ZERO ASSISTANCE
RESISTANCE
TRAINING

100% wheelchair-based workout program

by

Dan Highcock

Let's Tell Your Story Publishing

London

COPYRIGHT

Title: Zero Assistance Resistance Training: 100% wheelchair-based workout program

First published in 2016

Address: Let's Tell Your Story Publishing, 3 Century Court, Tolpits Lane, Watford, WD18 9RS

ISBN: 978-1-910600-06-1 (paperback version)

Book cover, interior design and editing: Colette Mason

ATTENTION

Dan Highcock accepts no liability for any injury, loss or damage resulting from physical exercise. By following his guide you voluntarily assume the inherent risk of physical / resistance training.

Should you suffer from any medical conditions, injuries or allergies, or should you be in any doubt whatsoever, you are advised to seek medical / professional advice before starting this program.

Any supplements featured within the plan are optional and must be taken in strict accordance with the manufacturer's recommendations. If in any doubt always consult a physician.

Always ensure your technique is correct, you train within your own capabilities and observe any safety practices / code of conducts present within your own gym.

Dan is a Genetic Supplements sponsored athlete.

Theraband® is a registered trademark of the Hygenic Intangible Property Holding Co.

*This book is dedicated to all the wheelchair users out there who say
a big "NO" to not getting it done, a big "NO" to not going out to get 'theirs,'
a big "NO" to not dominating their lives and
one last "NO " to the words "I CAN'T!"*

CONTENTS

ACKNOWLEDGEMENTS   12

FOREWORD   13

AUTHORS PREFACE   15

   ABOUT ME   15

   WHY I WROTE THIS BOOK   17

   HOW I CREATED THE PLAN   18

   HOW TO USE THIS BOOK   19

   STAYING MOTIVATED   19

INTRODUCTION   21

HOW THIS PROGRAM IS STRUCTURED   27

NUTRITION   31

   MACRONUTRIENTS   31

   MICRONUTRIENTS   32

   HOW TO CALCULATE YOUR TOTAL DAILY CALORIE NEEDS   33

   STORE CUPBOARD SHOPPING LIST   33

   DIETARY SUPPLEMENTS   39

THE PROGRAM   43

   BEFORE YOU START   44

   SCHEDULE   48

   MUSCLES   49

   TRAINING TECHNIQUES   52

PHASE 1

   SESSION A – DUMBBELLS ONLY   56

   SESSION B – CABLES ONLY   56

   SESSION C – CIRCUIT TRAINING (CABLE AND DUMBBELLS)   57

   SESSION D – SPEED / RECOVERY (RESISTANCE BANDS)   58

PHASE 2

   SESSION A – DUMBBELLS ONLY   60

   SESSION B – CABLES ONLY   60

   SESSION C – CIRCUIT TRAINING (CABLES AND DUMBBELLS)   61

   SESSION D – SPEED / RECOVERY (RESISTANCE BANDS)   62

PHASE 3

    SESSION A – DUMBBELLS ONLY   64

    SESSION B – CABLES ONLY   64

    SESSION C – CIRCUIT TRAINING (CABLES AND DUMBBELLS)   65

    SESSION D – SPEED / RECOVERY (RESISTANCE BANDS)   66

EXERCISES EXPLAINED   67

    BANDS   68

        BAND ALTERNATE HAND CHEST PRESS   68

        BAND ALTERNATE HAND SHOULDER PRESS   70

        BAND BICEP CURL   72

        BAND CHEST PRESS   74

        BAND EXTERNAL ROTATION   76

        BAND FACE PULLS   78

        BAND LAT RAISE   80

        BAND PULL APARTS   82

        BAND SHOULDER PRESS   84

        BAND TRICEP EXTENSION   86

    CABLES   88

        SINGLE-ARM CABLE CHEST PRESS   88

        SINGLE-ARM CABLE CURL   90

        SINGLE-ARM CABLE FRONT RAISE   92

        SINGLE-ARM CABLE LAT PULLDOWN   94

        SINGLE-ARM CABLE LAT RAISE   96

        SINGLE-ARM CABLE LOW ROW   98

        SINGLE-ARM CABLE REAR-DELT FLY   100

        SINGLE-ARM CABLE ROPE CURL   102

        SINGLE-ARM CABLE ROPE OVERHEAD EXTENSION   104

        SINGLE-ARM CABLE ROPE PUSHDOWN   106

        SINGLE-ARM CABLE ROW TO CHEST   108

        SINGLE-ARM CABLE SHOTGUN ROW   110

        SINGLE-ARM CABLE TRICEP EXTENSION   112

        SINGLE-ARM UNDERHAND GRIP PULLDOWN   114

    DUMBBELLS   116

        DUMBBELL CHEST PUNCHES   116

        DUMBBELL SHOULDER PUNCHES   118

        SINGLE-ARM ARNOLD PRESS   120

SINGLE-ARM BENT-OVER DUMBBELL RAISE   122

SINGLE-ARM CUBAN PRESS   124

SINGLE-ARM DUMBBELL EXTENSION   126

SINGLE-ARM DUMBBELL KICKBACK   128

SINGLE-ARM DUMBBELL LAT RAISE   130

SINGLE-ARM DUMBBELL ROW   132

SINGLE-ARM FARMER'S PUSH   134

SINGLE-ARM HAMMER CURL   136

SINGLE-ARM ROTATING CURL   138

SINGLE-ARM SHOULDER PRESS   140

PLATES   142

CROSSING PLATE PUNCHES   142

PLATE FIGURE 8S   144

REST AND RECOVERY   147

GLOSSARY   153

RESOURCES   157

KEEP IN TOUCH   157

ACKNOWLEDGEMENTS

Kerrie Louise Highcock – what can I say, my amazing wife. Thank you for all the support you give constantly and putting up with me when I'm grumpy, tired and stressed. Without your support I simply could not continue to achieve and do all the things that I am doing. Thank you x

Peter Jackson – my late grandfather and hero. Without this guy I simply would not be where I am today. I can't put into words what this man did for me when I was younger and for that I am – and will – be eternally grateful.

Colette Mason – this book would not be as good as it is without the help of Colette. She is not only my book coach but has also helped with various aspects of the it, including the front and back covers, editing, formatting and a whole host of other things. I know I've been a giant pain in the arse throughout, so Colette, thank you so much!

Michael Helbing – thank you for doing the photos for this book, free of charge I might add – very grateful for the help. Cheers!

Ian Patrick – thanks for being an eagle-eyed beta-reader and reviewer and helping me in the final stages.

Mike Samuels – thanks for stepping in and helping me with the back cover wording.

Joe Donnelly, Layne Norton, Elliott Hulse, Nick Mitchell – these 4 guys have been the main influences in my journey in the fitness world over the last 5 years. Thank you so much for inspiring me and enabling me to do what im doing now.

Richard Sennewald – my strength and conditioning coach. He's incredibly knowledgeable and has helped me tremendously over the past 12 months with my own specialised training for basketball.

Genetic Supplements – Thanks for supplying me with the highest quality products that enable me to keep at the top of my game.

All my friends and followers on social media – thank you for your continued support. You all know who you are.

FOREWORD

Rich Sennewald B.Sc. (Hons)

What Dan has put together in the following pages of this book is nothing short of fantastic – a compendium of training, nutrition and motivational tips and techniques designed but amazingly not limited to the wheelchair athlete.

Just being friends with and working with Dan has been rewarding enough and I'm thrilled to get to add a little flavour to the start of his book! He truly is an awe-inspiring athlete, I'm sure you'll agree once you've finished the first few chapters / sections.

As for Dan... 'the book' and where I fit in..?

I have worked with Dan for a long time now and it has been a fascinating experience. Through a lot of blood, sweat and tears, Dan and I sat down and studied countless movements to select appropriate lifts for supplementing basketball training in the sports and conditioning arena.

A real challenge that Dan has reflected on in the nutritional sections of the book is how we have found, through theory, trial and error, a differently-abled athlete eats.

Whilst we don't always agree on every principal (I'll still be holding onto my bagels), everything is soundly reasoned and has served Dan, large amount of his team mates and his clients very well in their pursuits.

It's also important to state that saying "they don't train as hard and require as much energy as a regular client due to immobility" – which has been an argument traditional thinkers have used in over simplifying coaching – is a ridiculous understatement.

Discussing activity levels and assessing energy requirements with Dan was an incredibly personal journey; any good nutritional coach can calculate energy uses of various activities and reflect that in a detailed plan. But, have you ever considered how exhausting moving on crutches is... or what the effect of an everyday life spent manoeuvring in a chair might be? The nutritional protocols Dan has settled on through our collaborations reflect this. They also reflect an understanding and appreciation many trainers don't possess – and would find it hard to get to grips with – having not experienced the physical "day-to-days" that Dan has. It's an area we'd love to work deeper in, to gather more accurate data for all athletes.

The training principals in the book are another fantastic experience we had. Traditional power generation movements for athletes transferring power through their lower limbs are out of the window. Creating high demand and effective cardiovascular training program, without the vast body of muscles of a fully able-bodied athlete has available to create a demand, was a tricky task as well.

It's amazing to see that Dan has essentially catalogued, archived and improved on all of this knowledge and presented it in the following pages. Of particular use will be the illustrated section, "Exercises explained" that will help also anyone coaching a wheelchair athlete.

Zero Assistance Resistance Training will no doubt see many, many prints, revisions and be developed further over time – because Dan is a perfectionist.

Enjoy this edition whilst it lasts!

Rich.

AUTHORS PREFACE

ABOUT ME

My name is Dan Highcock. I'm a 34-year-old Paralympic wheelchair basketball player and online personal trainer and nutrition coach.

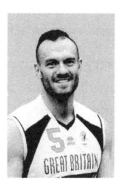

My story

At the age of 5, I had a motor bike accident, destroying my hip and pelvis, leaving me with a condition called *avascular necrosis* of the hip – a condition that worsens with age.

Sooner or later, I will be confined to a wheelchair full time – when, I'm not so sure. I needed hip surgery last year so the next problem may be the final problem. (But here's the thing, I have never let that thought ever make me too afraid to get out there and live life and try new things.)

After the accident, doctors and surgeons alike told my mother that I would never walk again. I was in hospital for over 6 months. This was followed by several more months at home in a full-body plaster cast.

Some of my earliest memories were being in school in my wheelchair, watching all the other kids playing football, running around and having fun. I wanted to do the same – but couldn't.

I remember at home, when my mum went out of the room, I would try to stand up and take steps around my chair, holding onto the side. I could barely put one foot in front of the other. If my mum had caught me, she would have gone crazy! As far as everyone was concerned, I was never walking again, end of story. All I know was that my consultant said any type of weight bearing was only going to make a bad situation even worse. What did he know, right?!

This was, and still is my mentality... screw what people say I can't do, if I want to do it, I sure as hell am going to!

This attitude progressed. At 13, I started using an exercise bike after school. I told my mum that I was involved in "after school clubs" but I didn't say what exactly – she would have gone nuts about that too if she found out the truth!

Very quickly, my legs got stronger and started to develop. It was around this time that I started to play wheelchair basketball.

In my chosen sport and in life in general, I have failed and been knocked down more times than I care to remember. But I don't let it stop me. I still have sporting and personal goals that I want to achieve. This is what keeps me going.

Every time I come out of the other side of failure and defeat, I learn a little more about myself and this strengthens my character. I also learn what I need to do differently next time.

"KEEP AWAY FROM PEOPLE WHO TRY TO BELITTLE YOUR AMBITIONS. SMALL PEOPLE ALWAYS DO THAT. BUT THE REALLY GREAT MAKE YOU FEEL THAT YOU TOO CAN BECOME GREAT."

MARK TWAIN

Thanks to my training and determination, I have played professional wheelchair basketball all over Europe, winning cups and titles both in the domestic leagues and domestic European Cups in the UK, Spain, Italy and Germany.

I have represented Great Britain in 3 world championships, 3 European championships winning 2 silver medals and 1 gold. I took part in the London 2012 Paralympics finishing in 4th place.

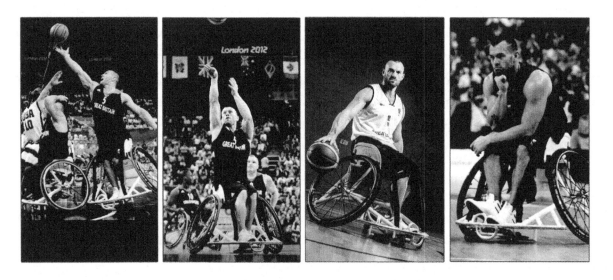

I am not telling you this to boast – I want to open your eyes to what's possible.

My attitude towards training is a no-nonsense, ball-busting style that will not only strengthen your body, but also your mind. Having the discipline and mind-set to go and push yourself to your absolute limits, way outside of your comfort zone, is great preparation for anything that life throws at you.

"WHEN YOU FEEL LIKE GIVING UP – YOU DON'T. YOU KEEP PUSHING ON AND COME OUT STRONGER ON THE OTHER SIDE."

DAN HIGHCOCK

What are you capable of achieving, I wonder? I would love to hear more about your progress.

WHY I WROTE THIS BOOK

I have spent countless hours over the years in the gym, working on my own performance. I've also written lots of different training and nutrition plans for my clients.

I noticed 1 particular problem for all my paraplegic, wheelchair-using clients – they all have varying levels of mobility and strength in their upper bodies. This meant some people could follow the plans I set out on their own. Others, had to rely on the help of a member of staff in the gym or a friend / training partner to help them complete the workouts.

Hiring a trainer for every session is a luxury most of us can't afford. Finding friends who can commit to 4 training sessions a week is difficult. We have to get on with it by ourselves. What's more, if you're fiercely independent like me, you want to be able to do things without help anyway.

This drove me to develop a complete training system that allows you to perform all exercises with ZERO ASSISTANCE from anyone else.

This 12-week plan works your whole upper body using only

- dumbbells
- plates
- adjustable cable rack
- resistance bands

HOW I CREATED THE PLAN

I have found you need to add a lot of variety to your workout to keep your body guessing. This is the best way to avoid the problem of your progress *plateauing*.

Over the years, I seen time and time again, it's best to use a range of

- training methods
- exercises
- repetitions
- rest times
- frequency

to get the best results. This approach varies the frequency, intensity, time-duration and type of exercise you do. (It's called the FITT principle... no pun intended ☺)

ENSURING IT'S SAFE AND IT WORKS

I've thoroughly tested this workout is safe. It can be done independently – you can *trust* it. Here's how I created it.

- used experience of what works in my own training sessions
- recalled how my clients liked to work
- came up with a draft routine
- tested each exercise can be done safely alone
- refined it
- tested it as a program with real people

Here's what one of my students said, Edward Joseph Molloy.

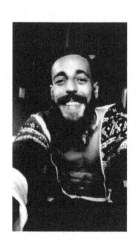

"Well what can I say! It's so nice to have someone fighting in our corner guys. ZART and this guy are undoubtedly worth your time and investment. ZART is easy to follow.

As a full-time wheelchair user and a qualified fitness instructor, I highly recommend buying this book. It will benefit your life beyond belief. The domino effect is real. Dan's book will leave you hoping for a sequel. It's so beneficial to anyone in a chair that has the need for more strength, mobility, fitness and independence. Highly recommended."

HOW TO USE THIS BOOK

To get the absolute best from this book, I suggest you read it through from start to finish, regardless of whether you are experienced in the gym or not. Let's have everything you are going to use fresh in your head. Anything that you don't understand, read through again until you do. Any technical terms in *italics* are listed in the glossary at the end of the book. This will give you a more in depth explanation with things like training terminology or anatomy and physiology terms.

STAYING MOTIVATED

From time to time, we all struggle with motivation – myself included. Here's a little tip I use with my clients when they are finding it hard to stay motivated.

Add an emotion to how you see your end result, so imagine

- how <u>great</u> you are going to feel when your day-to-day life becomes easier because of the physical and mental strength you have built
- how <u>accomplished</u> and <u>proud</u> you will feel when you see your physique changes and your numbers in the gym increase

This is what I use myself and I find it works great!

LOG YOUR PROGRESS

Be sure to download this extra bonus I have for you listed in the resources section!

It's a Zero Assistance Resistance Training workout log so you can input all your data from your workouts to see the improvements you make on a week-by-week basis.

WORK WITH ME

If you would like to find out a little more about working with me on a more personal, group or one-to-one basis, or just want to join me on social media, check out the "Keep in touch" section.

GETTING THE MOST OUT OF THIS PROGRAM

The biggest factors in determining your results are

- self-belief
- hard work
- consistency
- sacrifice
- patience

If you can master these 5 factors then you're on the road to success.

> "IF YOU CANT FLY, THEN RUN. IF YOU CANT RUN, THEN WALK. IF YOU CANT WALK, THEN CRAWL. BUT WHATEVER YOU DO, YOU HAVE TO KEEP MOVING FORWARD"
>
> MARTIN LUTHER KING JR

Dan Highcock
Personal trainer and nutrition coach
www.danhighcock.com
www.zar-training.com
September 2016

INTRODUCTION

Let's take a sneak peak at what we'll be learning together as you master the Zero Assistance Resistance Training (ZART) workout.

The beauty of this program is that it can be done with

- zero assistance
- 4 pieces of equipment only
- no need for transferring from your wheelchair to a bench or piece of equipment

HOW ZART WORKS

I mentioned earlier how varying your workout brings better benefits.

This chapter clearly explains the structure of the program and how it boosts your health and fitness. To make sure it's varied, it harnesses the power of 5 key training principles

- **strength training to boost your**
  - fitness level
  - immune system
  - ability to avoid injury
  - bone strength
  - joint stability
  - independence in daily life

- **hypertrophy training to boost**
  - the amount of muscle you have
  - metabolism which will in turn promote fat loss

- **conditioning training to boost**
  - cardiovascular health
  - recovery time

- **speed training to boost**
  - hand speed
  - force generated when lifting weights

Whilst training hard is important, it's also important to remember you need to give your body time to rest and recover between sessions. If you don't rest, you risk *overtraining*. This undermines the hard work you're putting in to improve your wellbeing. So, to make sure you get the best results, I've given you some advice about that – a 5th element to your training

- **recovery to boost your**
  - body's ability to repair itself and adapt
  - ability to avoid injury

NUTRITION

To fuel your exercise sessions and maintain your body, it's important eat correctly too. This chapter covers the main food groups, what they do for your body and the sort of foods to eat to boost your results. We'll start with macronutrients

- proteins
- carbohydrates
- fats
- fibre

Then we'll move onto micronutrients and some supplements you may wish to consider. (Supplements are a huge topic and could become a book on their own right, so I've opted to discuss the benefits of a few products that help most people with their training.)

- vitamins and minerals
- whey protein
- creatine

When it comes to how much to eat (what your calorific intake needs to be) I've provided 2 spreadsheets with simple calculations you can use to make sure you eat the right amount of food for your body's needs. These explain what you need to do to gain muscle or lose fat.

THE WORKOUTS

Once you understand the basics, it's time to focus on the workouts themselves.

ZART is a 12-week program consisting of

- 3 phases each lasting 4 weeks
- 4 different workout sessions per phase

This ensures there's plenty of variety, which keeps

- your body guessing to avoid plateauing
- your interest levels high – no one wants to do the same thing over and over again for 12 weeks solid – it gets dull

IMPORTANT: If you're new to exercise, pay attention to the advice in the "Before you start" section (see page 44,) to make sure you work out safely. It answers the common questions newbies ask me about how to train effectively.

EXERCISE DESCRIPTIONS

Each exercise has a concise explanation. Each description covers

- how to get into the start position
- how to perform the exercise repetitions safely
- how to finish

I mentioned earlier that people have different levels of mobility and strength in their upper bodies and it's common to need to modify things a little to suit your personal circumstances. Where possible, there are suggestions for different approaches to the same exercise so you can find a strategy that works for you. (Usually, the easiest thing to do is use lighter weights and bands so you retain good form throughout the movement.)

TIP: check out the controlling your bands and weights sections (see page 44) for some practical advice for getting in position and ready to start an exercise.

REST AND RECOVERY

Once you start exercising, it can be tempting to throw yourself completely into it. It's natural to want results and want them NOW. That said, it's important to remember that your body is not a machine. Just like a Formula 1 car needs to pull into the pit lane for new tyres to keep going, your body needs a "pit stop" to repair itself and get ready for the next session.

Recovery has 2 main approaches

- active recovery – doing light exercise to boost your ability to repair
- rest and recovery – things you can do to boost your general wellbeing

For active recovery, your recovery sessions will be performed on the same day as the speed sessions. This will be on last training day of the week and uses resistance bands.

For rest and recovery, we'll look at the role of

- sleep
- pre- and post-workout nutrition
- mobility and stretching
- self-massage

GLOSSARY

Some people reading this book will already be experienced at working out. For others it will be a new topic to explore.

I have avoided cramming the book with definitions and instead gathered them all together in the glossary at the end. This handy reference explains the terminology used. Remember, if you come across a term in *italics*, I've added it to the glossary for you.

RESOURCES

To help you stay on track and maximise your results, I have put together some additional resources for you. They help with tracking your workout progress and give you some suggestions for your food intake.

- 2 calorie intake needs calculators (1 for gaining muscle and 1 for losing fat)
- meal planner
- shopping list

- training planner workout log
- training methods crib sheet

You can download copies from my website and print them out. The resources section (see page 157) has more information.

KEEP IN TOUCH

My goal as your trainer is to make your workouts fun and effective. I am here to motivate you and help you get the results you deserve.

I'd love to hear from you about your experience with the ZART program. Do let me know how you feel about it. You can join my free Facebook group, "Feel, Look & Perform Amazing" and a special "ZART" group for you guys.

This section explains how to contact me. (See page 157.)

LET'S GET GOING

I'm super excited to show you all the things I have learnt and used not only with my clients but in my own training.

"LET'S DO THIS!!!!"

HOW THIS PROGRAM IS STRUCTURED

The Zero Assistance Resistance Training program has 5 key exercise components

- strength
- hypertrophy
- conditioning
- speed
- active recovery

It also includes an all-important rest and recovery component.

The exercise components are *periodised* into 4-week phases. Each one uses different exercises, methods, tempos and rest times in each phase, to stop things getting stale.

This means you maximise your overall potential because it prevents your progress from plateauing.

As well as boosting your results, the phases

- add variety to keep the sessions interesting, not monotonous
- introduce you to, and educate you in the use of different repetition (rep) ranges, methods and tempos
- reduce the chance of injury
- improve overall conditioning and cardiovascular health

TIP: If you're new to fitness, remember I have put together the getting started section with some advice for beginners, plus the glossary (see page 153) provides explanations of important terminology and concepts.

TRAINING PRINCIPLES

Let's look at the role each of the 4 training methods in detail and the benefits they bring.

STRENGTH

The clue is in the title with this! We are only using dumbbells for the strength sessions. This means your body has to engage a lot more muscles, such as your stabilising muscles, to perform these movements. We will be using heavy weights, low reps, slow, *eccentric* movements and explosive *concentric* movements.

HYPERTROPHY

Hypertrophy is the term used for muscle building. To get the best results for these sessions you will use a double or a single adjustable cable rack.

You will use moderate weight and slow speeds for each exercise, changing as we go through each phase. Here, the focus is contracting the exercised muscle as hard as possible, creating the best muscle pump we can. This causes little micro tears in the muscle due to all the blood in there, then the muscle will, with adequate nutrition and recovery, repair itself and grow back a little bit bigger. This is called *adaptation*.

CONDITIONING

This method improves your conditioning level – your body's ability to recover as fast as possible after intense bouts of exercise. This is achieved with circuit training.

Circuit training means performing several exercises back-to-back (a circuit) without rest. After the circuit, you get a brief rest period and then begin the next.

Because the circuits are taxing on your cardiovascular system (your heart, lungs and circulatory system) your heart rate will rise. What we are looking to improve on is how quickly your heart rate returns back to normal after the intense exercise you perform during the circuits. The quicker you heart rate gets back to normal, the fitter and healthier you are. Your general sense of wellbeing will be notably increased, I can assure you. You will just feel fantastic.

SPEED

Improving your speed levels, in particular your hand speed, enables you to generate more force, meaning over time, you can lift heavier. Also, if you play any sport, hand speed is always a great advantage to have.

You will train for speed using resistance bands only, performing specific movements for set periods of time using a 1-to-4 work to rest ratio.

These sessions are based on a brief period of intense activity followed by a longer rest period. For example, you perform the exercise repeatedly for 10 seconds as fast as you can, then rest for 40 seconds.

ACTIVE RECOVERY

Your active recovery sessions will be performed on the same day as the speed sessions on the last training day of the week, again, using resistance bands.

You will perform a warm-up prior (the bands component beforehand serves as a warm-up) to your speed work. You will do this again after your speed work. This will dramatically reduce the chances of injury. What's more, it will keep your shoulders healthy by working all the stabilising muscles at the rear of the shoulder. (These often get neglected, especially from using the front of the shoulders most of the time pushing the wheelchair around.)

SUMMARY

We've looked at how we maximise your results by varying the frequency, intensity, time and type of exercise you do.

I have explained the 5 main components of the program and the benefits you will gain

- strength
- hypertrophy
- conditioning
- speed
- active recovery

Next, we'll focus on nutrition and how you fuel your workouts.

NUTRITION

Nutrition is the biggest factor in seeing the "fruit of your labour" in the gym long term.

(I mean why go to all that effort if you're not going to fuel your body with the right nutrients in order to perform at your very best and to ensure optimal recovery?)

Let's start with a brief overview of the things that make up a balanced diet

- macronutrients
  - proteins
  - carbohydrates
  - fats
  - fibre
- micronutrients
  - vitamins
  - minerals

After that, we'll look at a sample shopping list what I always have in the fridge or cupboard at home. If you have these things in at all times, you will never be short of great, nutritious meals to eat.

MACRONUTRIENTS

Let's look at what macronutrients are and how they are used in the body. Then, I'll explain how to calculate how much you should be eating of each 1 using my downloadable spreadsheets.

PROTEINS

Protein has 4 calories per gram.

After water, the rest of the body is mainly made up of protein. Its main purpose is to build and repair tissue. As a rule of thumb, I suggest that you eat a good source of protein every 3 to 4 hours.

CARBOHYDRATES

Carbohydrate has 4 calories per gram.

Carbohydrates are the body's "go to" energy source. They are essential for great energy levels during long or intense periods of exercise. Your body also uses carbohydrates to replenish glycogen stores within your muscles, ensuring optimal recovery.

FATS

Fat has 9 calories per gram.

Although often demonised, fat is vital for the body. It is necessary to maintain healthy cell membranes, neurone function, the absorption of fat-soluble vitamins and hormone regulation and more.

FIBRE

Fibre is 2 calories per gram.

Fibres are complex carbohydrates that the body cannot digest in the same way as regular carbohydrates. They help to

- regulate blood sugar levels
- increase satiety making you feel fuller for longer
- reduce the risks of bowel disease and constipation

I suggest at least 30g per day but don't go higher than 60g.

MICRONUTRIENTS

VITAMINS AND MINERALS

These are essential in hundreds of metabolic processes, hormone production and lots of other things too. The list goes on and on!

All of these micronutrients can be found in fruit and vegetables. An easy way to make sure you meet your requirements is to eat plenty of colourful, natural foods daily.

(Note: I'll explain about whey protein and creatine in the supplements section.)

HOW TO CALCULATE YOUR TOTAL DAILY CALORIE NEEDS

As we are all genetically unique, we all need different amounts of the macronutrients I mentioned earlier. To find out how much you should be eating then please download my worksheets. (See the resources section on page 157 for details.) It works out all of the numbers for you quickly and easily. Remember to choose the gaining muscle or losing fat one, depending on your goals.

It is so important to track data when you have a goal in sight. You need to know your starting point and your end point. Simply guessing or going on how you feel in terms of nutrition is like driving blind. Your body is constantly adapting to the training and nutrition you're providing it with, so assessing your intake all the time is crucial for success.

For example, if you are trying to lose fat and you're maintaining your body fat level at 2,000 calories per day and you're not tracking what you're taking in, one day you might be in deficit and eat 1,800 calories. The next day you might eat too much, say 2,200 calories. You are no better off. You need to be precise. These type of situations occur frequently if you aren't tracking and measuring what you put into your mouth and leave it to guesswork.

> **TIP:** Although my spreadsheets are "one-size-fits-all" formulas, they work well. However, if you want to find out more about how I can help you create a bespoke, personalised nutrition program, visit my website. (See the keep in touch section on page 157.)

STORE CUPBOARD SHOPPING LIST

Below is a list of foods I like to keep at home. They are great for creating something quick, simple and nutritious, with minimal fuss.

It's best to stay clear of heavily processed foods. A lot of their nutritional content is lost, leaving you eating *empty calories*.

Let's look at what you should be eating, then I'll explain what to steer clear of. The best thing is not to buy any of the bad foods – then you can't feel tempted to eat them when you see them in the cupboard ☺.

PROTEIN OPTIONS	
RED MEAT	**POULTRY**
Salmon	Turkey
Beef	Chicken
Lamb	**WHITE FISH**
Veal	Dover sole
Venison	Prawns
Buffalo	Cod
Anchovies	Lobster
Duck	Crab
Pheasant	Haddock
Rabbit	**DAIRY**
Liver	Eggs
Kidney	Whey protein
DARK FISH	Milk
Sea bass	Cottage cheese
Mackerel	
Sardines	
Tuna	

VEGETABLE OPTIONS	
GREEN VEGETABLES	**ADDITIONAL VEGETABLES**
Broccoli	Peppers
Watercress	Tomatoes
Spinach	Onions
Cauliflower	
Green beans	
Kale	
Cabbage	
Brussels sprouts	
Asparagus	

(As fats are high in calories, I have added measures for portion sizes in the following tables to help you.)

FAT OPTIONS	
SOURCE	**10G FAT(APPROX)**
Coconut oil	10g (2 x teaspoons)
Butter	10g (2 x teaspoons)
Olive oil	10g (2 x teaspoons)
Nuts	12g
Nut butter	25g (5 x teaspoons)
Avocado	10g (1/2 an avocado is 50g)

CARBOHYDRATE OPTIONS	
SOURCE	**50G CARBOHYDRATE (APPROX)**
Sweet potato	250g (uncooked weight)
Brown rice	70g (uncooked weight)
Gluten-free oats	70g (uncooked weight)
Buckwheat pasta	70g (uncooked weight)
Quinoa	70g (uncooked weight)

DRINK OPTIONS	
SOURCE	**RESTRICTIONS (IF ANY) AND TARGET**
Filtered water	Any time – 4 litres
Green tea	Any time
Peppermint tea	Any time
Tulsi tea	Any time
Organic coffee	None after 16.00

VITAMINS AND MINERALS

You'll remember I said the easy way to ensure you're eating a wide range of vitamins and minerals is to eat plenty of different coloured, natural foods on a regular basis. The best sources are

- fruits
- vegetables

TIP: I recommend green vegetables like spinach and broccoli and berries such as raspberries, blueberries.

WHAT NOT TO EAT

The golden rule is to avoid heavily processed foods. There have been lots of scientific studies showing the harm caused to our bodies by eating too many processed foods. Obesity and an increased likelihood of cancer are 2 big reasons to cut down on your consumption.

Here is a list of things to <u>reduce</u> from your diet.

PROCESSED FOODS	
TYPE	**EXAMPLES**
Processed meat	Burgers (homemade are fine with lean steak mince) Sausages Sliced, packaged meat Shaped meat like chicken nuggets
Refined carbohydrates	Dried mashed potato White sugar, bread and pasta
Processed fats	*Trans fats* *Hydrogenated vegetable oil*

STAYING SANE

You'll notice I said <u>reduce</u> not <u>eliminate</u> from your diet. You need to be realistic. You will be tempted, fall off the wagon, go on holiday, work away from home, fancy a treat. The list goes on.

Here's my take on this. For me, life is all about balance. You need it or you will go crazy! Enjoy the things you love, just don't binge – BE MINDFUL!

I use the 80 / 20 rule. That means, if you eat well **80%** of the time, your body can manage the other 20%. That said, if your goal is very specific and has a time constraint, then you may want to eat as well as possible all the time.

CHOOSE SINGLE INGREDIENT FOODS ALL THE WAY

You'll notice, all my store cupboard foods are simple, single ingredient foods – that means they are made up of 1 thing.

You've probably noticed as foods become more processed, the ingredients list on the packaging gets longer and longer! Some processed foods so many additives, the ingredients list looks more like a paragraph in a chemistry book than a cookbook.

As a rule of thumb, if any particular food has an ingredient that you cannot easily pronounce, then stay clear for maximal health benefits.

The easiest thing is to stick to simple, single ingredient foods. When you make a meal, you do the "adding" not the food processing factory!

And of course, don't have bad foods in the house – you have to put in a lot more effort to go out and buy some when tempted, so it makes it much easier to stay committed.

ALCOHOL

There is room for alcohol in your lifestyle. As I mentioned earlier, you need balance. Again, though, it may hinder you hitting your goal if there is a tight deadline looming, or you simply want to improve as fast as possible.

Alcohol has 7 calories per gram so it's pretty calorie dense. And they are all empty!

> **TIP:** I recommend swapping your calories from alcohol for the calories you would normally consume from either carbohydrates, fats or a combination of both.

So this means, if your plan is to consume 2,000 calories a day, and you drank 500 calories worth of alcohol, now you have 1500 calories to consume in the form of food. You would have to reduce your carbohydrate or fat intake by 500 calories, or say, 250 calories from each.

I highly recommend hitting your protein intake as normal. Don't be tempted to reduce that.

Again, try not to keep alcohol at home to reduce cravings.

> **TIP:** Never binge drink! This really will slow down your progress.

CHEAT MEALS

Now you see I didn't say CHEAT DAY! A cheat MEAL. Having a full-on cheat day can easily undo all the hard work you have put in over the previous week. People tend to go crazy.

In actual fact, I HATE the words "CHEAT MEAL" too!

If you are tracking your foods and know what your daily intake of calories and macros is then you can make the "cheat meal" fit in at any time. Remember the 80 / 20 rule I stated before.

> **TIP:** If you would like to know more about flexible dieting and the "If It Fits Your Macros" (IIFYM) diet check out the keep in touch section on page 157.

FALLING OFF THE WAGON

It's very (very!) easy and very common for people to "fall off the wagon," both in terms of training and nutrition. Here's how to deal with it.

If you have a bad day eating or you miss the gym for whatever reason, it's usually because life gets in the way, right? For everyone, it's the same. Don't go into "f**k it mode" and go crazy. If you slip up, dust yourself off, compose yourself, realise what's just happened and "get back on the wagon" ASAP!

In the grand scheme, 1 bad day here and there won't affect your long-term results, but 3, 4, 5 bad days in a row, regularly sure as hell will!

DIETARY SUPPLEMENTS

If you have a balanced diet, you're well on the way to meeting all your requirements. If you are following a very intense program (I work out twice a day as a pro-athlete), or are reducing your calorie intake to lose fat, supplements can be a real bonus.

Here is a short list of recommended supplements to take whilst on the training program. There is a wide range of supplements I could recommend but everyone has a different budget to spend on such items (if any budget at all) so I'm keeping my list to 2 key items for now. If you want some personalised advice, just ask.

> **TIP:** For most people, taking supplements is not essential. Eating well is enough. Remember, if you are taking medication, check that there will be no adverse side-effects.

WHEY PROTEIN

This has to be the daddy of all sports nutrition supplementation. It is the fastest digesting and most rapidly absorbing protein source making it a clear favourite with gym goers and pro-athletes alike.

Whey comes in 2 forms

- isolates
- concentrate

If you are *lactose intolerant* stick with whey isolates as the lactose levels are extremely low.

I recommend 30 to 40 grams of whey protein post-workout. This is going to be digested the quickest and therefore set to work the quickest on repairing the muscles after your gym sessions. You can also use *protein shakes* to help you hit your daily protein targets.

It is best taken post-workout. That said, if you forget, or you're on a rest day, you could still have some in order to hit your daily protein needs.

CREATINE

Creatine is probably the most-studied sport supplement over the past 20 years.

It allows the body to perform at higher levels of intensity for longer periods of time. There are so many types of creatine products on the market, it can be a little confusing. *Creatine monohydrate* is all that's needed.

You DO NOT need 1 of the more expensive ones and you most certainly DO NOT need to do a *loading phase*. Five grams in your post workout shake is sufficient.

SUMMARY

We've looked at the role of eating properly in your success. We started by looking at the main food groups and the role in nutrition.

- macronutrients
  - proteins
  - carbohydrates
  - fats
  - fibre

- micronutrients
  - vitamins
  - minerals

You've seen a list of healthy things I like to keep in my store cupboard and things you should avoid. I also gave you some tips on how to eat well and how to handle things not going to plan.

We finished off with a brief look at a couple of supplements

- whey protein
- creatine

Now you know how to have a varied training plan and how to fuel your workouts, it's time to turn our attention to the how to work out safely and effectively during the 3 core phases of your 12-week plan.

THE PROGRAM

In this section, I'll begin with some advice on how to follow the program safely and effectively. We'll cover

- **what you need to know before you start**
    - how to control your bands and weights
    - how to keep yourself stable
    - how to look after your spine
    - how to keep good form
    - how to keep breathing
    - the importance of tensing your muscles mid-exercise
    - how to protect your joints
- **hints and tips**
    - dealing with pre-existing injuries
    - how to plan your workouts
    - modifying exercises
- **the training schedule**
    - when to work out
    - what session sequence to follow
- **an explanation of the training techniques**
    - repetitions (reps)
    - sets
    - supersets
    - circuits
    - 15 method
    - 28 method
    - tempos for reps

Once you know the ropes, we'll go through the 3 phases and discover the 4 workouts that make up each 1.

BEFORE YOU START

Work out safely! Getting injured isn't fun, slows you down and worst case, can cause long-term or permanent damage. It's important to read the instructions on how to perform a rep for each of the exercises safely.

CONTROLLING YOUR BANDS AND WEIGHTS

I want to share some ideas for the most ergonomic and straightforward ways to get in position.

DUMBBELL AND PLATE TIPS

- when picking up dumbbells always hold onto 1 side of your wheelchair or the rack for stability BEFORE lifting your chosen dumbbell off the rack
- bend at waist while keeping your back straight as you pick up dumbbells with the palms of your hands facing each other
- keep weights on your lap else place them on a bench next to you for easy access
- keep your chair's brakes on while performing the exercises

BANDS TIPS

- bands can be tied to your chair's frame or wheels, a nearby bench or anything else sturdy that you can attach it to in order to perform the exercises
- buy a range of different coloured bands (these are markers for how much resistance there is in each band) since you are going to get stronger whilst on ZART and will need to increase the resistance in the bands
- buy 2 of each band to save you the trouble of tying and untying every time you switch sides
- you can wheel on top of the band instead of attaching it to something for some exercises (remember to apply brakes)
- you can use bands with or without handles
- if your strength levels aren't so great right now, it may be a good idea to start off using Theraband® branded bands instead – there will be less resistance

STABILITY

- always have you brakes on
- hold on to your frame with the opposite hand that you are performing the exercise with or hold onto a bench when it's in the incline position

KEEP YOUR SPINE NEUTRAL

A neutral spine means keeping your spine held straight (and still retaining its light natural curve) as you exercise. Think of it as sitting up proud with good posture.

Whatever angle you might be leaning at, you keep your back held in the same "good posture" pose. Try to keep a neutral spine as much as possible through each exercise. This may mean lifting less weight than you think you can handle. I realise this may be more challenging for some than others but just work within your limits.

KEEP GOOD FORM

It's important to learn to do each exercise correctly. This is called "good form." The better your form, the less likely you are to hurt yourself. It also means better results. If you're struggling to maintain good form you have 2 options

- decrease the weight you're using
- reduce number of repetitions

Remember that proper form matters whenever you use weights. This includes when you pick up and replace your weights on the racks.

KEEP BREATHING

As you concentrate on the exercise, you might be tempted to hold your breath while you're lifting weights. Keep breathing and never hold your breath. When you hold your breath, you build up your carbon dioxide in your body which will cause you to fatigue faster.

Holding your breath as you handle the resistance from the weight can affect how your blood circulates in your chest and dramatically raise your blood pressure.

There's a simple way to avoid this. Get into the habit of breathing in as you "work" with a weight and inhale as you return to the more relaxed start position.

KEEP THE WORKING MUSCLE UNDER CONSTANT TENSION

To get the best results you should keep the working muscle under constant tension from start to finish in every rep you perform, in each set. Doing this ensures that the stress is being placed upon the main muscle and not the smaller supporting muscles or joints. This also maximises the training benefits, which are building muscle and getting stronger.

DON'T FULLY LOCK YOUR JOINTS

When you are doing an exercise and you fully extend your arms until they can't straighten anymore, it becomes "locked" in place.

This takes tension off the working muscle (see above) which is what we don't want.

At best, locking your joints gives your muscles a rest at the halfway point, making your session less effective. It's a form of cheating.

At worst, if you're holding weights and have locked elbows, it places an enormous amount of stress on the joint, instead of working your muscles. This can lead to joint problems and / or injury.

People instinctively bend their knees as they land after jumping to deal with resistance and avoid injury. Think of this when trying to remind yourself not to lock your elbows.

HINTS AND TIPS FOR ZART

If you're new to exercise, you've probably got a lot of questions. Here's the most common things I get asked.

Can I move the workout schedule around?

Yes, if you need to. But ZART has been put together to give adequate rest (48 hours) between training overlapping muscle groups. Try to avoid training the same body parts on consecutive days. It's important to recover if you want to maximise your results.

I have injured body part X, can I still train it?

I would advise NO – do not train it and seek the advice of a doctor or relevantly qualified medical professional for a diagnosis and treatment. If you choose to train on it regardless, no one is going to stop you – but a full blown injury may well do! Use common sense.

It's important for me to point out that you are going to be sore from these workouts. This post-exercise soreness does not mean you are injured – it's a phenomenon called delayed onset muscle soreness (DOMS.) It's quite normal. It's that moderate ache that develops over time after you do something a little bit more physical than your body is used to. You tend to feel it the next day when you wake up, never during the workout.

I can't do exercise Y (due to lack of equipment or discomfort.) What can I do instead?

For some of the exercises I have provided modifications. If you find these are not appropriate for your own circumstances, please contact me at dan@zar-training.com and let's work out an alternative together.

SCHEDULE

Phases 1, 2 and 3 all follow the same daily schedule. Please note that although this can be adjusted to suit your personal daily life schedule, the plan I put here in example 1 is the most optimal. If you do need to change days, you should do the workouts in the same order of A, B, C and D. Don't have more than 2 days back-to-back with workouts. Give your body time to rest.

Example 1

This plan shows you how you could change the days of the week you work out on and still follow the sequence and rest day recommendations.

	MON	TUES	WED	THURS	FRI	SAT	SUN	OK?
Phase 1	A	B		C	D			☑
Phase 2	A		B		C	D		☑
Phase 3			A	B		C	D	☑

Example 2

This plan won't work as there are 2 sets of 3-day workouts without rest in phases 1 and 2. In phase 3, the order has been changed *and* the rest is insufficient.

	MON	TUES	WED	THURS	FRI	SAT	SUN	OK?
Phase 1	A		B			C	D	☒
Phase 2	A				B	C	D	☒
Phase 3	A	D				C	B	☒

MUSCLES

To be the strongest, fittest and healthiest as possible then we need to stay injury free and have complete balance in terms of front (anterior) & back (posterior) muscle groups.

As I'm sure most of you are well aware, a very common problem faced by wheelchair users is that they can be really rounded in the shoulders. This is because they spend the majority of the time pushing forwards, developing the front shoulder muscles (deltoids) and hardly any time balancing that out by doing pulling movements.

This can lead to all sorts of problems such as shoulder impingements. Trust me, I've had my share of shoulder problems so I make it non-negotiable that I do the correct amount of pushing to pulling movements. This is a "pre-hab" strategy which is built into your ZART program.

FRONT VIEW

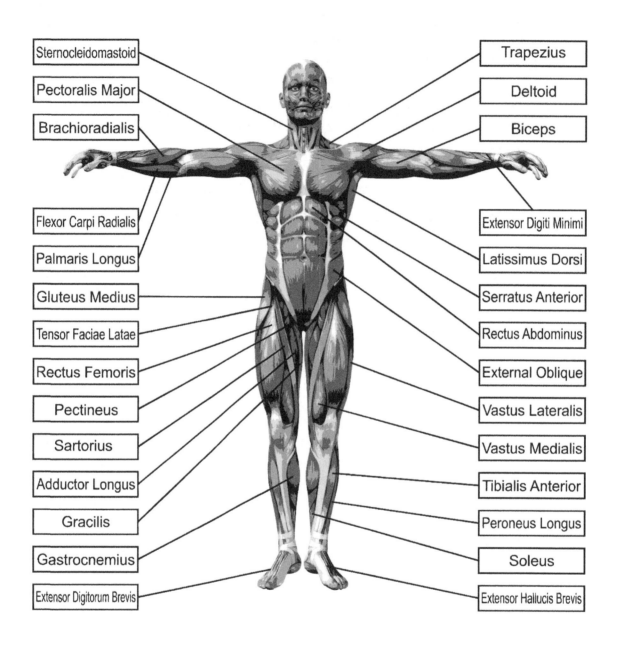

Sternocleidomastoid

Pectoralis Major

Brachioradialis

Flexor Carpi Radialis

Palmaris Longus

Gluteus Medius

Tensor Faciae Latae

Rectus Femoris

Pectineus

Sartorius

Adductor Longus

Gracilis

Gastrocnemius

Extensor Digitorum Brevis

Trapezius

Deltoid

Biceps

Extensor Digiti Minimi

Latissimus Dorsi

Serratus Anterior

Rectus Abdominus

External Oblique

Vastus Lateralis

Vastus Medialis

Tibialis Anterior

Peroneus Longus

Soleus

Extensor Hallucis Brevis

BACK VIEW

Trapezius

Deltoid

Rhomboid

Teres Major

Triceps

Extensor Carpi Radialis

Extensor Carpi Ulnaris

Extensor digitorum

Extensor Digiti Minimi

Latissimus Dorsi

Thoraco-lumbar Fascia

Gluteus Maximus

Gracilis

Vastus Lateralis

Semimembranosus

Semitendinosis

Biceps Femoris

Gastrocnemius

Soleus

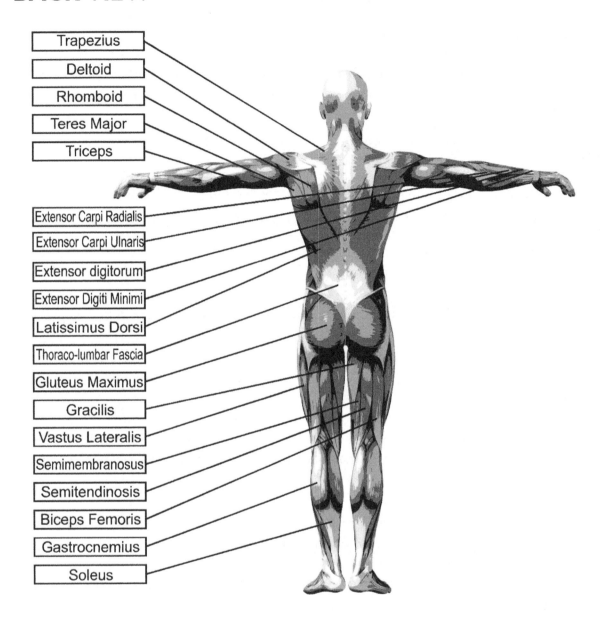

TRAINING TECHNIQUES

REPETITIONS (REPS)

Repetitions are normally referred to as "reps." A rep is the actual movement phase of each exercise. For example, for a dumbbell curl, curling the dumbbell up and then lowering the dumbbell back down is 1 repetition.

SETS

Every time you perform a certain number of reps, for example 10, that is one set. When you see 4x10 written in the workouts it means 4 sets of 10 reps – i.e. number of sets x number of reps.

SUPERSET

This is doing 2 sets of exercises back-to-back without rest. This is counted as 1 superset. Supersets are great for creating a great muscle pump, necessary for hypertrophy and also great for cardiovascular conditioning.

CIRCUITS

Each exercise in the circuit workout list is to be performed back-to-back without rest until the list is completed. Once the list is complete, you get a rest before starting the next circuit.

Circuits are good for increasing cardiovascular conditioning as you are performing long bouts of high-intensity exercise followed by short rest times.

Circuits never get easier as you get fitter – you just work harder. (I can assure you, the more conditioned you are, the more of an arse-kicker in life, in general you will be.)

Start off with 3 circuits and see how it goes. Work your way up to five.

15 METHOD

Choose a weight you can just about get 10 reps with, then the remaining 5 just perform the "flexion" part of the rep, i.e. for a

- bicep curl, it's the top half of the rep
- tricep pushdown, it's the bottom half of the rep

28 METHOD

- 7 reps regular speed
- 7 super slow reps
- 7 reps performing the first half of the rep only
- 7 reps performing the second half of the rep only

Lift around 30% of what you can normally as this is really hard.

TEMPOS

Most of the time in the workouts you will see 3-0 or 4-0 tempo. This means the amount of time it takes to do each rep.

The first number is the negative part of the rep, for example lowering the dumbbell on a bicep curl. The second number is the positive part of the rep, i.e. the lifting of the dumbbell on a bicep curl..

Let's look at some examples

3-1-1-1	3-second negative • 1 second hold at bottom • 1 second positive or "lift" • 1 second hold at top
0 (zero)	No pauses • perform the rep as normal with no pauses
4-0-X-0	Explosive (X) • four second lowering then straight back up as hard and as fast as possible

PHASE 1

WEEKS 1 TO 4

SESSION A – DUMBBELLS ONLY

ID	EXERCISE	SETS	REPS	TEMPO	REST
1	Single-arm Cuban press	4	8	4-0-X-0	90 secs
2	Single-arm dumbbell row	4	8	4-0-X-0	90 secs
3	Single-arm hammer curl	4	8	4-0-X-0	90 secs
4	Single-arm dumbbell extension	4	8	4-0-X-0	90 secs

SESSION B – CABLES ONLY

ID	EXERCISE	SETS	REPS	TEMPO	REST
1	Single-arm cable chest press	4	12	3-0-3-0	60 secs
2	Single-arm cable rear-delt fly	4	12	3-0-3-0	60 secs
3	Single-arm cable lat pulldown	4	12	3-0-3-0	60 secs
4	Single-arm cable curl	4	12	3-0-3-0	60 secs
5	Single-arm rope pushdown	4	12	3-0-3-0	60 secs

SESSION C – CIRCUIT TRAINING (CABLE AND DUMBBELLS)

ID	EXERCISE	SETS	REPS	TEMPO	REST
1	Single-arm shoulder press	3-5	8	1-0-X-0	3 mins after all 7 exercises are complete
2	Single-arm cable chest press	3-5	8	1-0-X-0	
3	Single-arm cable row to chest	3-5	8	1-0-X-0	
4	Single-arm dumbbell lat raise	3-5	8	1-0-X-0	
5	Single-arm rotating curl	3-5	8	1-0-X-0	
6	Single-arm dumbbell kickback	3-5	8	1-0-X-0	
7	Single-arm farmer's push (10-20 metres each arm)	3-5	8	X	

SESSION D – SPEED / RECOVERY (RESISTANCE BANDS)

ID	EXERCISE	SETS	REPS	TEMPO	REST
1	Band pull aparts	3	10	2-0-2-0	20 secs
2	Band external rotation	3	10	2-0-2-0	20 secs
3	Band face pulls	3	10	2-0-2-0	20 secs
4	Band alternate hand chest press (20 secs duration)	4	1	X	80 secs
5	Band shoulder press (20 secs duration)	4	1	X	80 secs
6	*Superset* Band tricep extension / bicep curl (20 secs duration)	4	1	X	80 secs

PHASE 2

WEEKS 5 TO 8

SESSION A – DUMBBELLS ONLY

ID	EXERCISE	SETS	REPS	TEMPO	REST
1	Single-arm Arnold press	4	6	4-0-X-0	90 secs
2	Single-arm dumbbell row	4	6	4-0-X-0	90 secs
3	Single-arm rotating curl	4	6	4-0-X-0	90 secs
4	Single-arm dumbbell extension	4	6	4-0-X-0	90 secs

SESSION B – CABLES ONLY

ID	EXERCISE	SETS	REPS	TEMPO	REST
1	Single-arm cable chest press	4	15	15 method	60 secs
2	Single-arm cable low row	4	15	15 method	60 secs
3	Single-arm cable lat raise	4	15	15 method	60 secs
4	Single-arm rope curl	4	15	15 method	60 secs
5	Single-arm cable tricep extension	4	15	15 method	60 secs

SESSION C – CIRCUIT TRAINING (CABLES AND DUMBBELLS)

ID	EXERCISE	SETS	REPS	TEMPO	REST
1	Single-arm cable chest press	3-5	12	1-0-X-0	2 mins after 1 circuit of all 7 exercises
2	Single-arm Arnold press	3-5	12	1-0-X-0	
3	Single-arm cable shotgun row	3-5	12	1-0-X-0	
4	Single-arm bent-over dumbbell raise	3-5	12	1-0-X-0	
5	Plate figure 8s	3-5	12	1-0-X-0	
6	Single-arm underhand grip pulldown	3-5	12	1-0-X-0	
7	Single-arm farmer's push (10-20 metres each arm)	3-5	12	X	

SESSION D – SPEED / RECOVERY (RESISTANCE BANDS)

ID	EXERCISE	SETS	REPS	TEMPO	REST
1	Band pull aparts	3	10	2-0-2-0	20 secs
2	Band external rotation	3	10	2-0-2-0	20 secs
3	Band face pulls	3	10	2-0-2-0	20 secs
4	Band chest press (10 secs duration)	4	1	X	40 secs
5	Band alternate hand shoulder press (10 secs duration)	4	1	X	40 secs
6	Band lat raise (10 secs duration)	4	1	X	40 secs

PHASE 3

WEEKS 9 TO 12

SESSION A – DUMBBELLS ONLY

ID	EXERCISE	Sets	Reps	Tempo	Rest
1	Single-arm shoulder press	4	4	4-0-X-0	90 secs
2	Single-arm dumbbell row	4	4	4-0-X-0	90 secs
3	Single-arm hammer curl	4	4	4-0-X-0	90 secs
4	Single-arm dumbbell extension	4	4	4-0-X-0	90 secs

SESSION B – CABLES ONLY

ID	EXERCISE	SETS	REPS	TEMPO	REST
1	Single-arm cable chest press	3	28	28 method	60 secs
2	Single-arm underhand grip pulldown	3	28	28 method	60 secs
3	Single-arm cable front raise	3	28	28 method	60 secs
4	Single-arm rope overhead extension	3	28	28 method	60 secs
5	Single-arm cable curl	3	28	28 method	60 secs

SESSION C – CIRCUIT TRAINING (CABLES AND DUMBBELLS)

ID	EXERCISE	SETS	REPS	TEMPO	REST
1	Dumbbell shoulder punches	3-5	20 secs	X	60 secs after 1 circuit of all 7 exercises
2	Dumbbell chest punches	3-5	20 secs	X	
3	Plate figure 8s	3-5	20 secs	X	
4	Single-arm hammer curl	3-5	20 secs	X	
5	Single-arm dumbbell kickback	3-5	20 secs	X	
6	Crossing plate punches	3-5	20 secs	X	
7	Band pull aparts	3-5	30 secs	X	

SESSION D – SPEED / RECOVERY (RESISTANCE BANDS)

ID	EXERCISE	SETS	REPS	TEMPO	REST
1	Band pull aparts	3	10	2-0-2-0	20 secs
2	Band external rotation	3	10	2-0-2-0	20 secs
3	Band face pulls	3	10	2-0-2-0	20 secs
4	*Superset* Band shoulder press / chest press (5 seconds duration)	4	1	X	20 secs
5	*Superset* Band bicep curl / tricep extension (5 seconds duration)	4	1	X	20 secs

EXERCISES

EXPLAINED

BANDS

BAND ALTERNATE HAND CHEST PRESS

Setup	1. secure bands around bar of pulley machine or a post at chest height
	2. test band is secure
	3. set appropriate tension
	4. sit facing away from pulley
Start	5. grab both band ends or handles
	6. position handles close to shoulders
	7. rotate wrist forward so palm faces forward
Rep motion	8. exhale and press left handle forward
	9. inhale and press right handle forward, returning left hand to start position at the same time
	10. complete reps stated in worksheet
End	11. replace bands

Tips

✓ the photo shows you how to position the band

Start / End

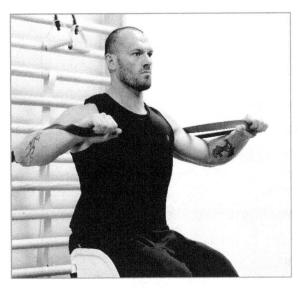

Alternate position 1

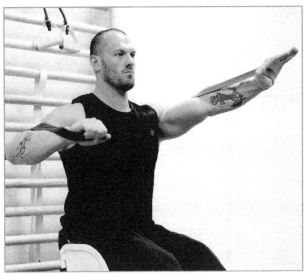

Alternate position 2

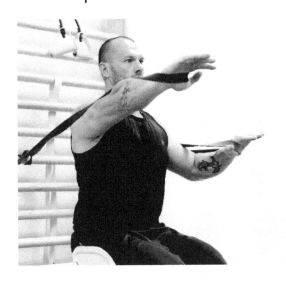

BAND ALTERNATE HAND SHOULDER PRESS

Setup	1. wheel onto band and apply brakes
	2. test band is secure
	3. set appropriate tension so it begins at arm's length
Start	4. grasp band in each hand and lift, so both hands are at shoulder height
	5. rotate wrists so palms face forwards
	6. bend elbows, keeping upper arms and forearms in
Rep motion	7. exhale and extend left hand upwards
	8. inhale and press right handle forward, returning left hand to start position at the same time
	9. complete reps stated in worksheet
End	10. release tension off band
	11. replace bands

Start / End

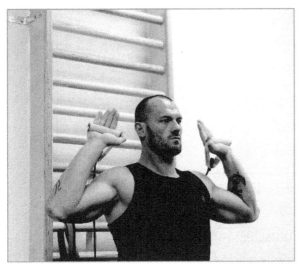

Alternate position 1

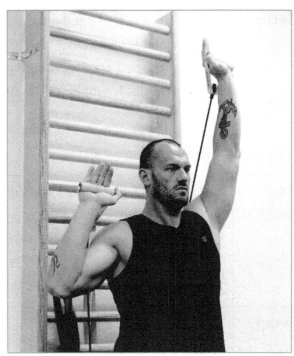

Alternate position 2

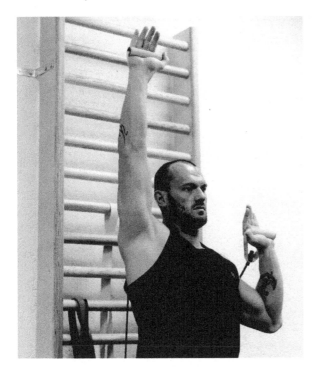

BAND BICEP CURL

Setup	1. wheel on top of band and apply brakes
	2. test band is secure
	3. set appropriate tension with arms at arm's length
	4. left arm holds wheel for stability
Start	5. keep upper arm is still, perpendicular to floor with elbows in and palms facing forwards
Rep motion	6. exhale and slowly curl arm upwards, keeping upper arm still until forearm touches your bicep
	7. pause for a second and squeeze muscles
	8. inhale and lower arm down to start position
	9. complete reps stated in worksheet
Swap	10. release tension off band
	11. complete reps for other arm
End	12. replace bands

Start / End

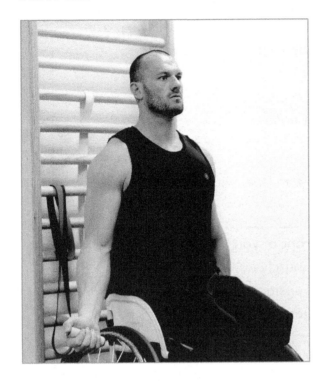

Position 1

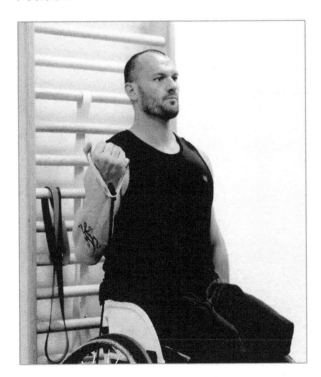

BAND CHEST PRESS

Setup	1. attach centre of band to a still object such as cable pulley bar at chest heigh (or simply put it around your upper back)
	2. test band is secure
	3. set appropriate tension for both arms
	4. sit with back to band attachment point
Start	5. hold one end in each hand
	6. bend elbows and position upper arm level with shoulder so hands are next to chest
Rep motion	7. exhale and extend arms out in front of you
	8. pause for a second and squeeze muscles
	9. inhale and slowly return to start position
	10. complete reps stated in worksheet
End	11. release tension off band
	12. replace bands

Tips

✓ remember to adjust resistance by wrapping band round your hand

Start / End

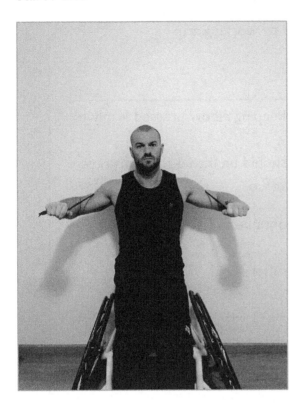

Position1

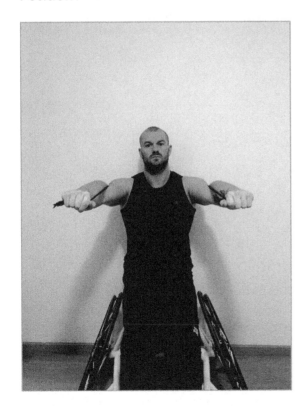

BAND EXTERNAL ROTATION

Setup	1. attach band around opposite wheel to working arm
	2. test band is secure
	3. set appropriate tension
Start	4. grasp end of band with right hand, keeping elbow pressed firmly to torso
	5. with upper arm in position, elbow should be flexed to 90 degrees with hand reaching across front of torso
Rep motion	6. rotate arm in a backhand motion continue as far as able, keeping elbow still
	7. hold for 1 second at contracted position
	8. complete reps stated in worksheet
Swap	9. release tension off band
	10. complete reps for other arm
End	11. replace bands

Start / End

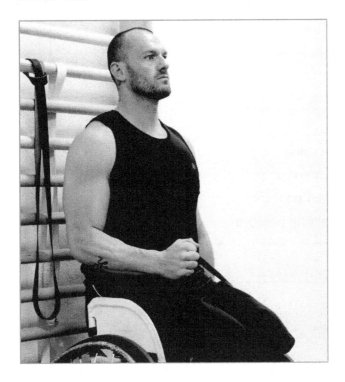

Position 1

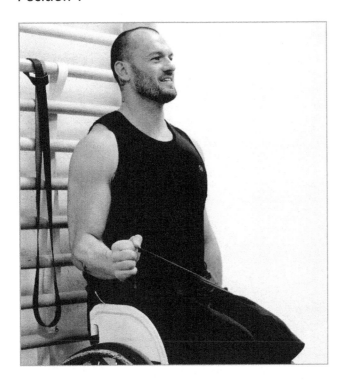

BAND FACE PULLS

Setup	1. attach band to a high position on either a post or the cable pulley
	2. sit far away enough so that you have good tension on the bands
	3. apply brakes
Start	4. sit with neutral spine
Rep motion	5. keep upper arms parallel to ground
	6. exhale and pull band directly towards face, separating hands
	7. hold for 1 second at contracted position
	8. inhale and return hands to starting position
End	9. replace bands

Start / End

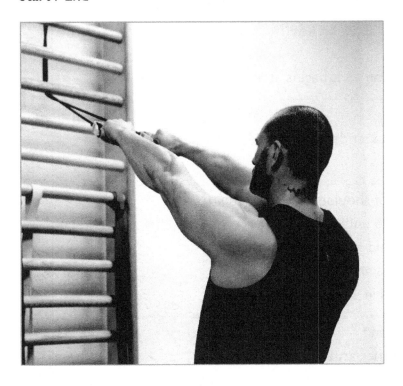

Position 1

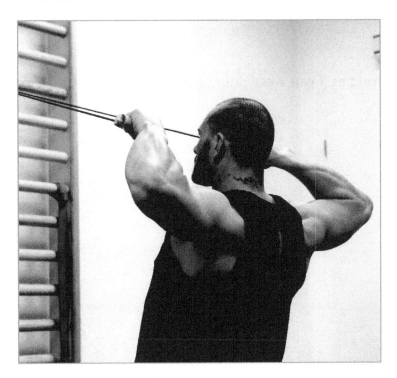

BAND LAT RAISE

Setup	1. wheel onto band and apply brakes 2. test band is secure 3. set appropriate tension so it begins at arm's length
Start	4. keep a neutral spine 5. grasp band and rest extended arm on sides of wheel, palms facing inwards
Rep motion	6. exhale and use side of shoulders to lift handle to side 7. continue to lift handle until shoulder height 8. pause for a second and squeeze muscles 9. inhale and return to start position 10. complete reps stated in worksheet
Swap	11. release tension off band 12. complete reps for other arm
End	13. replace bands

Tips

- ✓ as you lift handle, slightly tilt hand as if you were pouring water and keep your arms extended.
- ✓ keep your torso still

Start / End

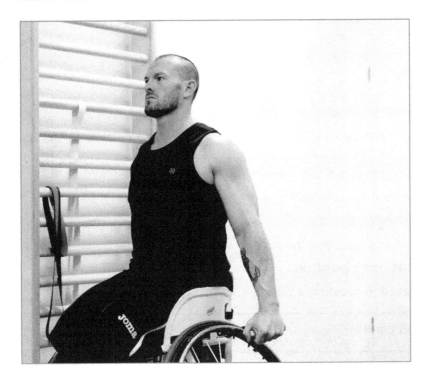

Position 1

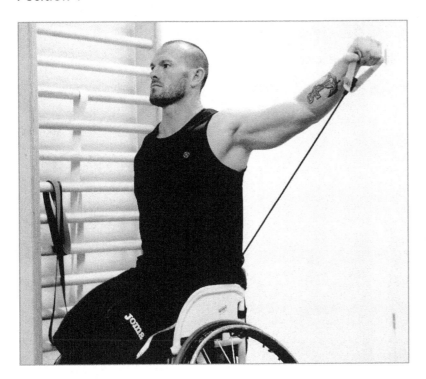

BAND PULL APARTS

Setup	1. select band position
	2. test band is secure
	3. set appropriate tension
Start	4. begin with both arms extended straight out in front, each holding a band end shoulder width apart
Rep motion	5. move hands out laterally to sides (reverse fly position)
	6. keep elbows extended as you perform movement
	7. bring band to starting position
	8. pause for a second and squeeze muscles
	9. inhale and return to start position
	10. complete reps stated in worksheet
Swap	11. release tension off band
End	12. replace bands

Tips

✓ keep your shoulders back during exercise

Start / End

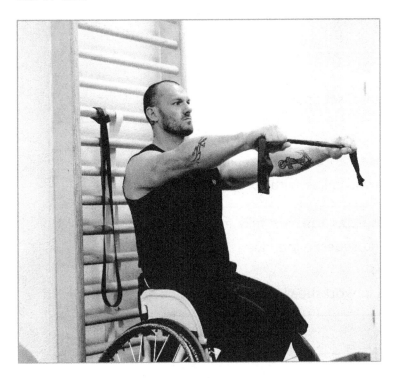

Position 1

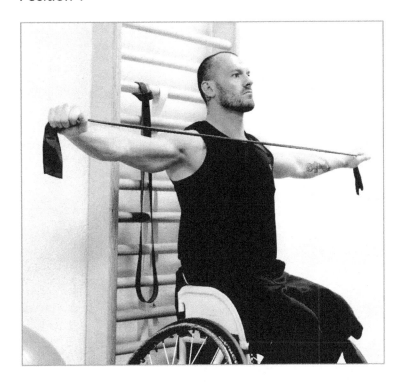

BAND SHOULDER PRESS

Setup	1. wheel on top of band
	2. apply brakes
	3. test band is secure
	4. with arms down by sides, set appropriate tension
Start	5. grasp and lift both handles to shoulder height
	6. rotate wrists so palms face forwards, keeping elbows bent, with upper arms and forearms in line with torso
Rep motion	7. exhale and lift handles up as arms are fully extended overhead
	8. pause for 1 second and squeeze muscles
	9. inhale and lower arms
	10. complete reps stated in worksheet
End	11. replace bands

Start / End

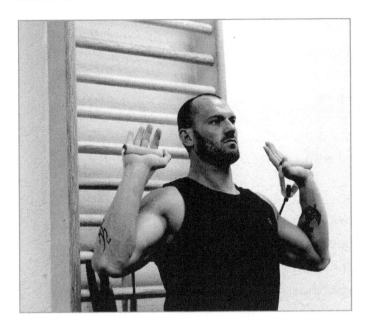

Position 1

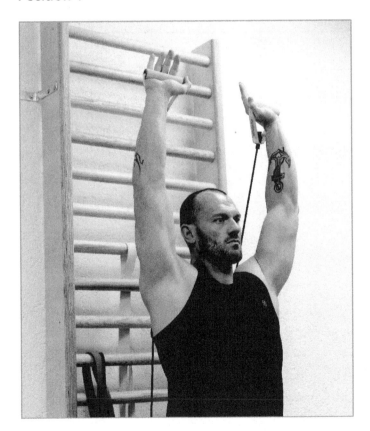

BAND TRICEP EXTENSION

Setup	1. wheel on top of band and apply brakes
	2. test band is secure
	3. set appropriate tension (arm position tension)
	4. sit upright with a neutral spine
Start	5. grab wheel with non-lifting hand
	6. pull right band behind head with elbows upwards, palms facing upwards
Rep motion	7. exhale and straighten elbow, keeping torso still
	8. pause for 1 second and squeeze muscles
	9. inhale and return to start position
	10. complete reps stated in worksheet
Swap	11. release tension off band
	12. complete reps for other arm
End	13. replace bands

Start / End

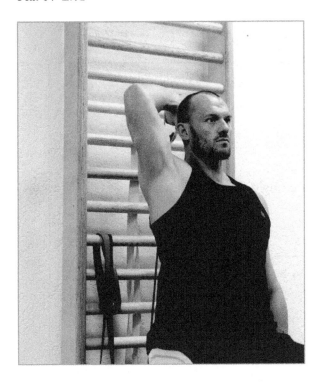

Position 1

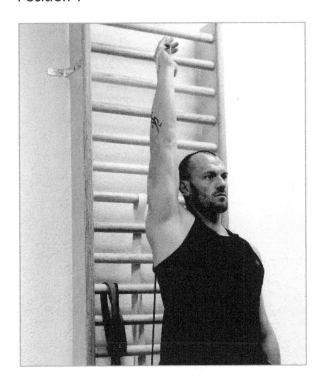

CABLES

SINGLE-ARM CABLE CHEST PRESS

Setup	1. set pulley to chest height and select appropriate weight 2. attach D-ring handle 3. sit 30 to 60cm in front of cable
Start	4. hold handle in right hand 5. position upper arm at a 90-degree angle with shoulder blades together 6. keep a neutral spine
Rep motion	7. exhale and extend elbow to press handle forward and in front of you, keeping rest of body still 8. pause for 1 second and squeeze muscles 9. inhale and return to start position 10. complete reps stated in worksheet
Swap	11. slowly lower cable and return weight onto stack 12. swap hands and complete reps for other arm
End	13. return weight to stack

Tips

✓ remember to keep your torso still and maintain a neutral spine
✓ you can stagger way you sit for better stability

Modifications

• if you are struggling to control the weight, try using a lighter 1

Start / End

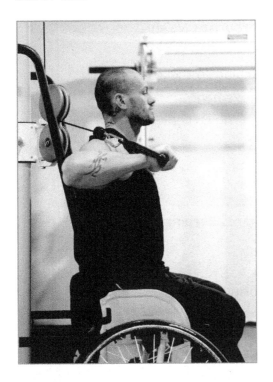

Position 1

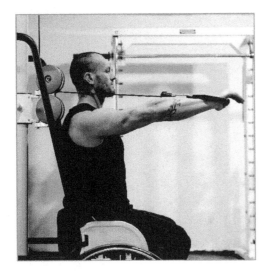

SINGLE-ARM CABLE CURL

Setup	1. set pulley to low position and select appropriate weight
	2. attach D ring handle
	3. grasp D ring, sitting far enough from machine so there is constant muscle tension throughout the whole movement
Start	4. keep upper arm still, perpendicular to floor with elbow in and palm forwards
	5. grasp chair with right arm to keep balance
Rep motion	6. exhale and slowly curl single handle upwards keeping upper arm still until forearm touches bicep
	7. pause for a second and squeeze muscles
	8. inhale and lower handle back to start position
	9. complete reps stated in worksheet
Swap	10. slowly lower cable and return weight onto stack
	11. swap hands and complete reps for other arm
End	12. return weight to stack

Tips

✓ remember to only move your forearm

Start / End

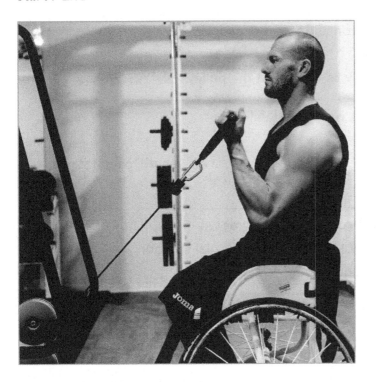

Position 1

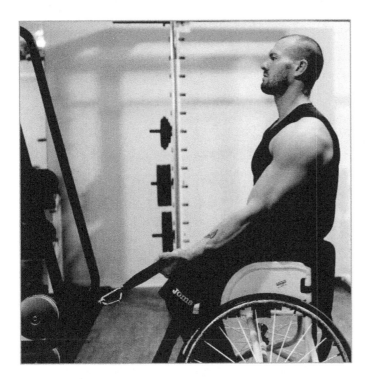

SINGLE-ARM CABLE FRONT RAISE

Setup	1. set pulley to lower position and select appropriate weight
	2. attach single handle
	3. sit facing away and slightly to the left of the pulley
Start	4. hold onto wheel with left hand for stability
	5. keep a neutral spine
	6. hold handle in right hand at side of wheel at arms' length, palm facing behind
Rep motion	7. exhale and raise arm to front, palm facing down
	8. continue to raise arm until slightly above parallel to floor
	9. pause for 1 second and squeeze muscles
	10. inhale and return to start position
	11. complete reps stated in worksheet
Swap	12. slowly lower cable and return weight onto stack
	13. reposition chair to slightly to the right of the cable pulley and swap hands and complete reps for other arm
End	14. return weight to stack

Tips

✓ remember to avoid locking elbows

Start / End

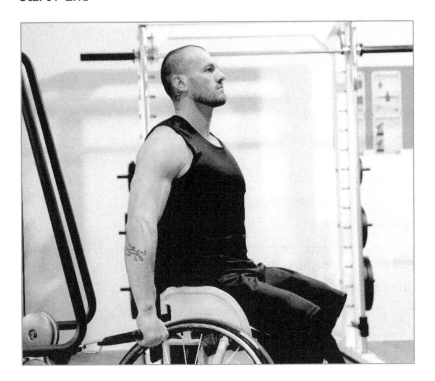

Position 1

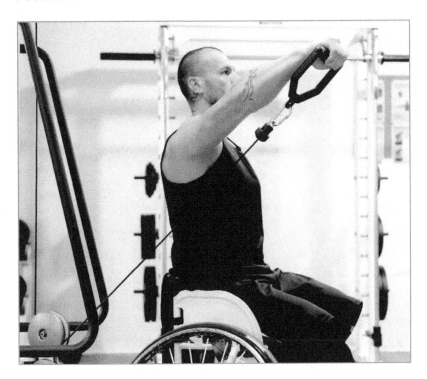

SINGLE-ARM CABLE LAT PULLDOWN

Setup	set pulley to high position and select appropriate weight attach D ring handle sit 30 to 60cm in front of cable
Start	grasp handle with left hand, palm inwards
Rep motion	exhale and pull handle down pause for 1 second and squeeze muscles inhale and return handle to start position complete reps stated in worksheet
Swap	slowly lower cable and return weight onto stack . swap hands and complete reps for other arm
End	. return weight to stack

Tips

✓ remember to keep some tension on your muscles as you return to start position
✓ pinch shoulder blades back first, then pull

Start / End

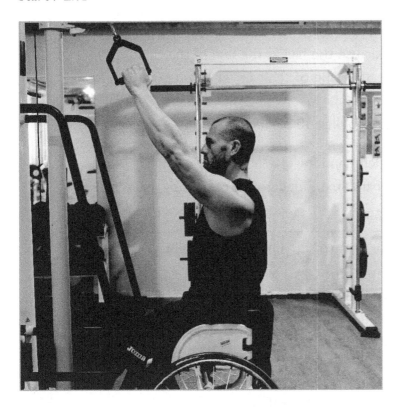

Position 1

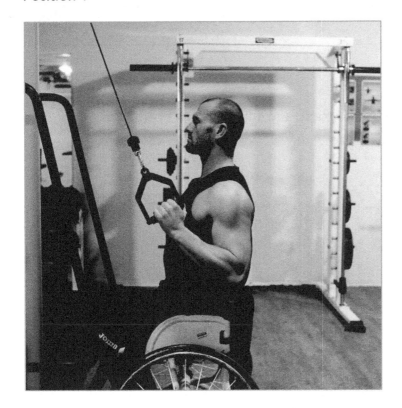

SINGLE-ARM CABLE LAT RAISE

Setup	1. set pulley to lower position and select appropriate weight
	2. attach D ring handle or use the ball at the end of the cable
	3. let cable run underneath frame of chair or let it run slightly in front of knees
	4. sit with left side next to pulley 30 to 60cm away
Start	5. hold onto chair with left hand for stability
	6. grasp handle in right hand, extended arm across body, palm facing towards body
Rep motion	7. exhale and raise upper arm to side until it is parallel to floor at shoulder height
	8. pause for 1 second and squeeze muscles
	9. inhale as you lower arm to start position
	10. complete reps stated in worksheet
Swap	11. slowly lower cable and return weight onto stack
	12. swap hands and complete reps for other arm
End	13. return weight to stack

Tips

✓ maintain upper arm perpendicular to torso and a fixed elbow position (10 degree to 30 degree angle) throughout exercise

Start / End

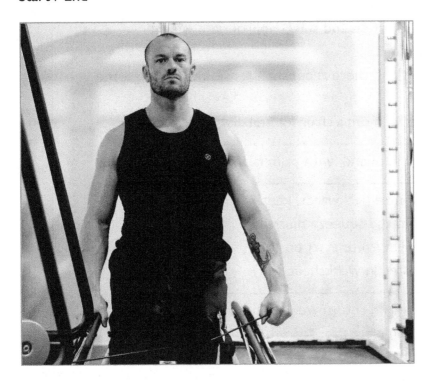

Position 1

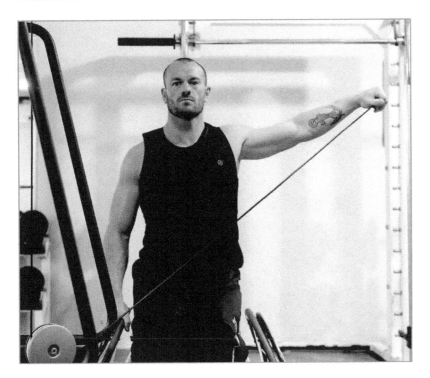

SINGLE-ARM CABLE LOW ROW

Setup	1. set pulley to low position and select appropriate weight
	2. attach single handle
	3. sit far away enough so there is constant tension throughout the movement
	4. use right hand to hold onto chair for stability
Start	5. grasp handle with left hand with palm facing inwards
Rep motion	6. exhale and pull handle backwards, keeping arms in
	7. pause for a second and squeeze muscles
	8. inhale and slowly return to start position
	9. complete reps stated in worksheet
Swap	10. slowly lower cable and return weight onto stack
	11. swap hands and complete reps for other arm
End	12. return weight to stack

Start / End

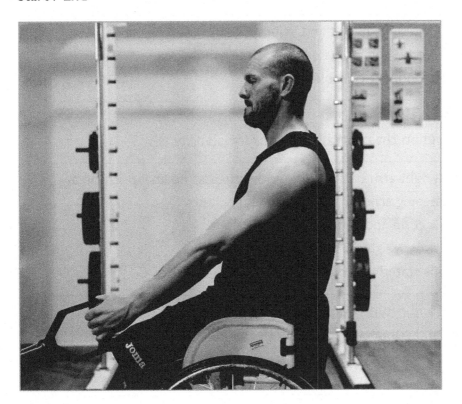

Position 1

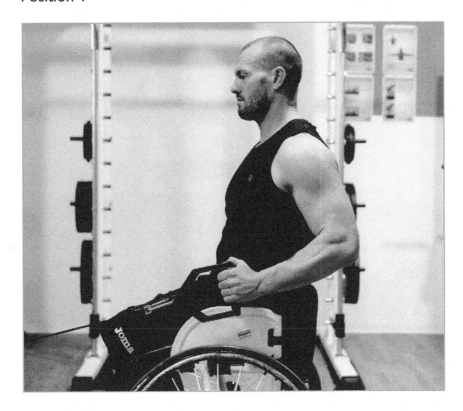

SINGLE-ARM CABLE REAR-DELT FLY

Setup	1. set pulley to shoulder height and select appropriate weight
	2. use the ball on the end of the cable as the "handle"
	3. sit 30 to 60cm in front of cable
Start	4. grasp handle in right hand
	5. place left hand on chair or cable rack or for stability
Rep motion	6. grip ball, pull right arm back until it goes just past normal position at shoulders, keeping arm long and elbow unlocked
	7. pause for 1 second and squeeze muscles
	8. inhale and lower weight back to start position
	9. complete reps stated in worksheet
Swap	10. return cable and return weight onto stack
	11. swap hands and complete reps for other arm
End	12. return weight to stack

Start / End

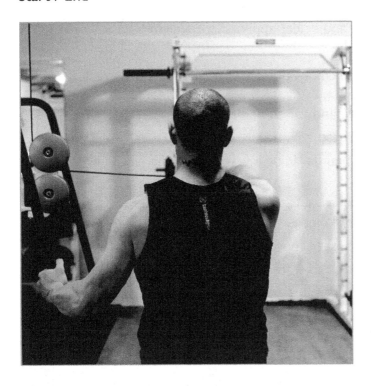

Position 1

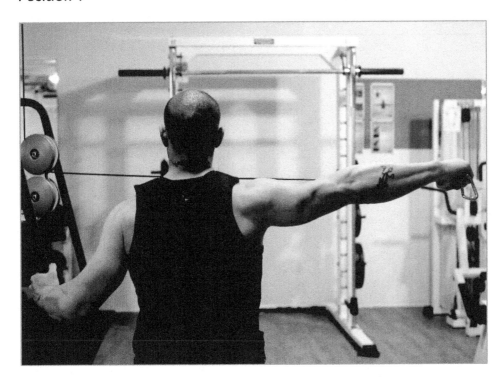

SINGLE-ARM CABLE ROPE CURL

Setup	1. set pulley to low position and select appropriate weight
	2. attach rope handle
	3. sit facing machine about 30 cm away from it to the left of the pulley
Start	4. hold onto chair with right hand for stability
	5. keep a neutral spine and torso still
	6. grasp rope with left hand, palms facing inwards, keeping elbow in during entire movement
Rep motion	7. exhale and raise handle until biceps touch forearm
	8. pause for 1 second and squeeze muscles
	9. inhale and lower handle back to start position
	10. complete reps stated in worksheet
Swap	11. slowly lower cable and return weight onto stack
	12. reposition chair and swap hands
	13. complete reps for other arm
End	14. return weight to stack

Tips

- ✓ remember only forearm should move
- ✓ keep your upper arm still

Start / End

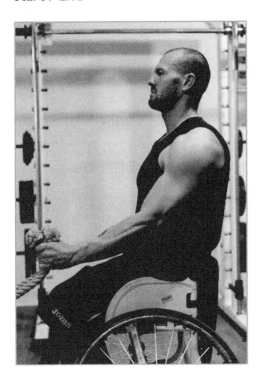

Position 1

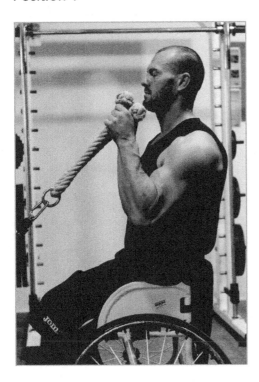

SINGLE-ARM CABLE ROPE OVERHEAD EXTENSION

Setup	1. set pulley to lower position and select appropriate weight
	2. sit close to the cable pulley, around 20 to 30cm away
Start	3. grab wheel with non-lifting hand for stability
	4. grasp rope with the other hand, extending arm until hand directly above head, palm facing inwards
	5. keep elbow close to head and arm perpendicular to floor, pointing knuckles at ceiling.
Rep motion	6. exhale and lower cable behind head, keeping upper arms still
	7. pause for a second and squeeze muscles
	8. inhale and return to start position, feeling stretch on triceps
	9. complete reps stated in worksheet
Swap	10. slowly lower cable and return weight onto stack
	11. swap hands and complete reps for other arm
End	12. return weight to stack

Start / End

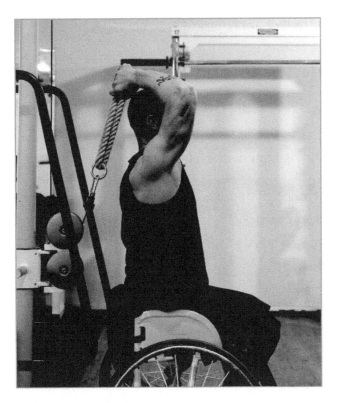

Position 1

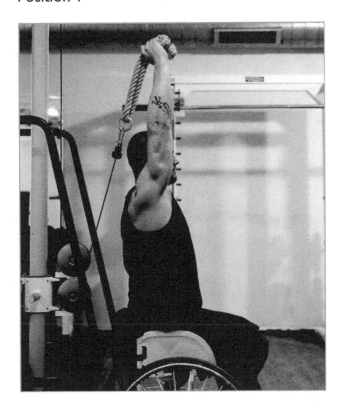

SINGLE-ARM CABLE ROPE PUSHDOWN

Setup	1. set pulley to high position and select appropriate weight
	2. attach rope handle
	3. sit 30 to 60cm in front of cable
Start	4. sit upright with torso straight
	5. bring upper arm close to torso and perpendicular to floor
	6. point forearm upwards as it holds rope with neutral grip
Rep motion	7. exhale and straighten elbow to bring rope down towards hips
	8. hold for 1 second at contracted position
	9. inhale and bring rope slowly up to start position
	10. complete reps stated in worksheet
Swap	11. slowly lower cable and return weight onto stack
	12. swap hands and complete reps for other arm
End	13. return weight to stack

Tips

- ✓ remember upper arm should always remain still next to your torso
- ✓ only forearm should move

Start / End

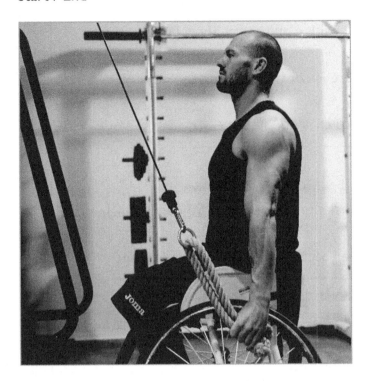

Position 1

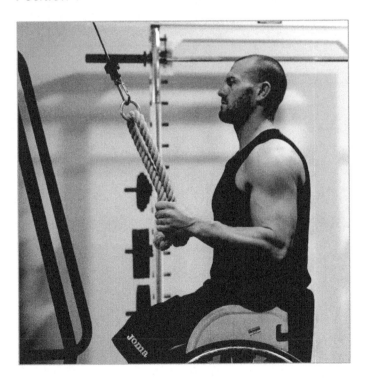

SINGLE-ARM CABLE ROW TO CHEST

Setup	1. set pulley to chest height position and select appropriate weight 2. attach single handle 3. sit far away enough so there is constant tension throughout movement 4. use right hand to hold onto chair for stability
Start	5. keep a neutral spine 6. grasp handle with left hand with palm facing down 7. with arm extended, pull back until torso is at a 90-degree angle from legs 8. notice light stretch in upper back as you hold handle in front
Rep motion	9. exhale and pull handle backwards, keeping arms in 10. pause for a second and squeeze muscles 11. inhale and slowly return to start position 12. complete reps stated in worksheet
Swap	13. slowly lower cable and return weight onto stack 14. swap hands and complete reps for other arm
End	15. return weight to stack

Start / End

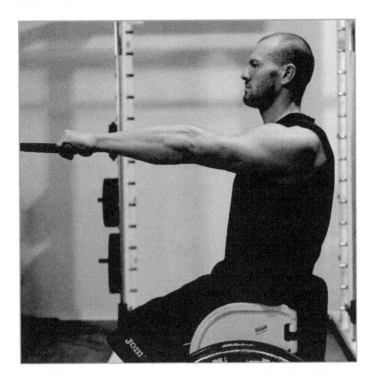

Position 1

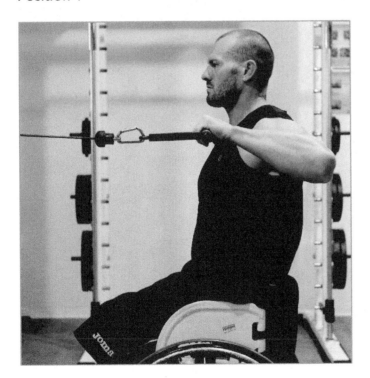

SINGLE-ARM CABLE SHOTGUN ROW

Setup	1. set pulley to low position and select appropriate weight
	2. attach single handle
	3. sit 60 cm away facing towards pulley
Start	4. grasp handle with left hand, palm facing inwards
	5. extend arm with shoulder facing forwards
Rep motion	6. exhale and bend elbow and lower upper arm, slowly turning palm upwards
	7. pause for a second and squeeze muscles
	8. inhale and return to start position
	9. complete reps stated in worksheet
Swap	10. slowly lower cable and return weight onto stack
	11. swap hands and complete reps for other arm
End	12. return weight to stack

Start / End

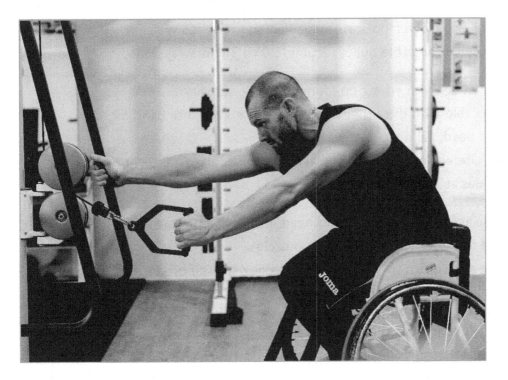

Position 1

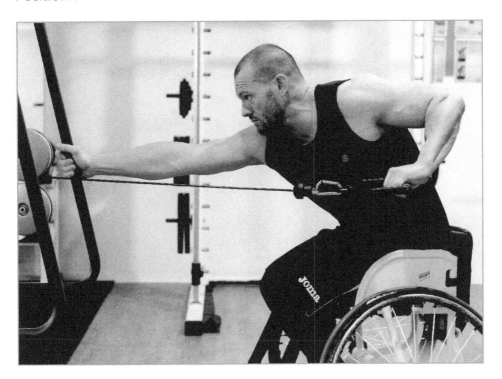

SINGLE-ARM CABLE TRICEP EXTENSION

Setup	1. set pulley to lower position and select appropriate weight 2. sit close to the cable pulley, around 20 to 30cm away
Start	3. grasp wheel with your non-lifting hand for stability 4. grasp cable with the other hand, extending arm until hand directly above head, palm facing inwards 5. keep elbow close to head and arm perpendicular to floor, pointing knuckles at ceiling
Rep motion	6. exhale and lower cable behind head, keeping upper arms still 7. pause for 1 second and squeeze muscles 8. inhale and return to start position, feeling stretch on triceps 9. complete reps stated in worksheet
Swap	10. slowly lower cable and return weight onto stack 11. swap hands and complete reps for other arm
End	12. return weight to stack

Start / End

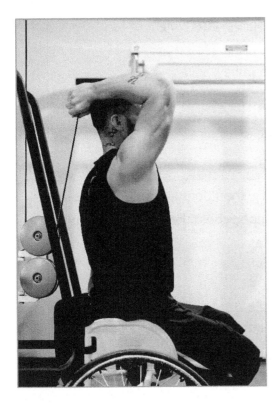

Position 1

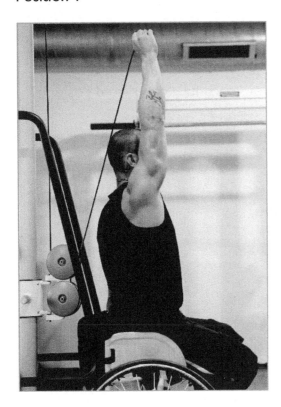

SINGLE-ARM UNDERHAND GRIP PULLDOWN

Setup	1. set pulley to top position and select appropriate weight
	2. attach D ring handle
	3. sit in front slightly to the right of cable pulley
Start	4. keep a neutral spine
	5. grasp D ring with left hand, palm facing inwards
	6. lean torso back slightly
Rep motion	7. exhale and pull D ring down by drawing shoulders and upper arms down and back until handle touches upper chest, keeping elbows in
	8. pause for a second and squeeze muscles
	9. inhale and return to start position
	10. complete reps stated in worksheet
Swap	11. slowly lower cable and return weight onto stack
	12. swap hands and complete reps for right arm
End	13. return weight to stack

Tips

- ✓ remember to hold onto wheel with non-lifting hand for stability
- ✓ concentrate on squeezing back muscles once you reach fully contracted position
- ✓ keep elbows close to your body
- ✓ upper torso should remain still as your bring handle towards you
- ✓ keep your torso still thoughout

Start / End

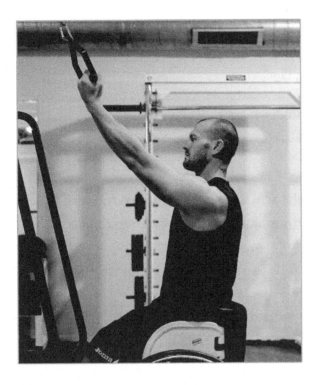

Position 1

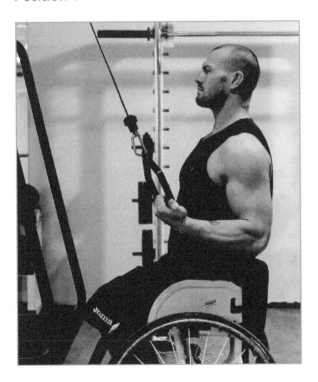

DUMBBELLS

DUMBBELL CHEST PUNCHES

Setup	1. pick up 2 dumbbells and place on lap
Start	1. grasp dumbbells and bring to shoulder height 2. rotate wrist with palms facing inwards
Rep motion	3. keep a neutral spine 4. exhale and explosively extend right arm until fully extended forwards 5. return right hand to shoulder and simultaneously begin to extend left fully forwards 6. maintaining control, swap arm positions as quickly and explosively as possible 7. complete time duration stated in worksheet
End	8. place dumbbells on lap for next exercise or replace on rack

Start / End

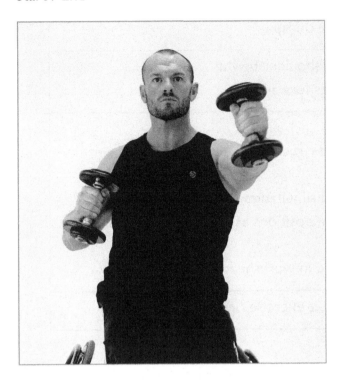

Position 1

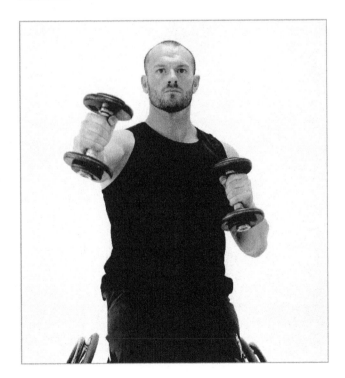

DUMBBELL SHOULDER PUNCHES

Setup	1. pick up 2 dumbbells and place on lap
Start	2. grasp dumbbells and bring to shoulder height 3. rotate wrist so that palm faces forwards
Rep motion	4. keep a neutral spine 5. exhale and explosively extend right arm until fully extended overhead 6. begin to lower right hand and simultaneously begin to raise right 7. maintaining control, swap arm positions as quickly and explosively as possible 8. complete time duration stated in worksheet
End	9. place dumbbells on lap for next exercise or replace on rack

Tips

- ✓ choose light dumbbells weighing 1kg to 5kg
- ✓ keep your torso still
- ✓ remember to keep breathing

Start / End

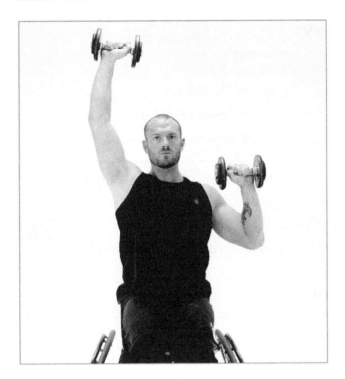

Position 1

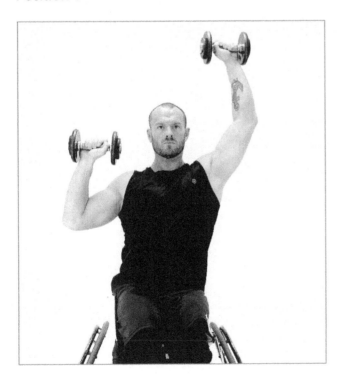

SINGLE-ARM ARNOLD PRESS

Setup	1. pick up dumbbell and place on lap
Start	1. keep a neutral spine 2. hold onto wheel with left hand 3. grasp dumbbell in right hand and raise it in front at upper chest level with palm facing torso, keeping elbows slightly bent
Rep motion	4. exhale and raise dumbbell by extending arm until weight is above head, turning your wrist to face forwards 5. pause for a second and squeeze muscles 6. inhale and lower dumbbell to start position, rotating palm towards torso 7. complete reps stated in worksheet
Swap	8. rest dumbbell on lap and swap hands 9. complete reps for other arm
End	10. place dumbbell on lap for next exercise or replace on rack

Start / End

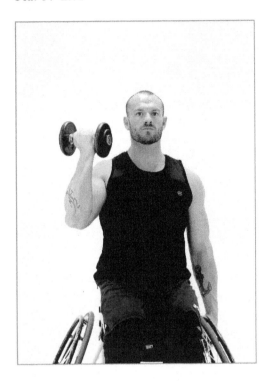

Position 1

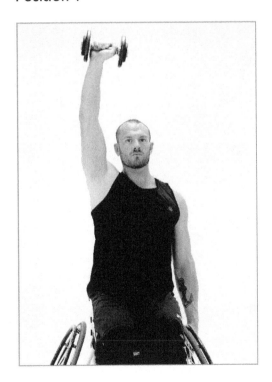

SINGLE-ARM BENT-OVER DUMBBELL RAISE

Setup	1. pick up dumbbell and place on lap
Start	2. keep a neutral spine
Rep motion	3. exhale and lift dumbbell upwards and outwards until arm is parallel to floor, keeping torso still 4. pause for 1 second and squeeze muscles 5. inhale and return to start position 6. complete reps stated in worksheet
Swap	7. rest dumbbell on lap and swap hands 8. complete reps for other arm
End	9. place dumbbells on lap for next exercise or replace on rack

Tips

- ✓ remember not to swing, keep still
- ✓ avoid locking elbows

Start / End

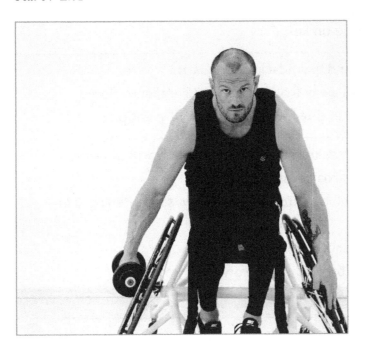

Position 1

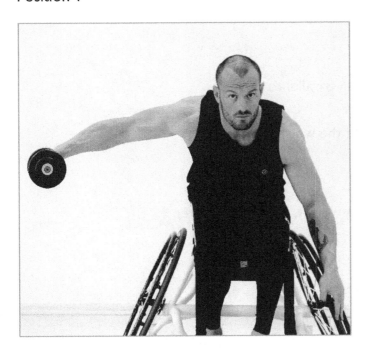

SINGLE-ARM CUBAN PRESS

Setup	1. pick up dumbbell and place on lap
Start	2. take dumbbell in right hand, palm facing backwards 3. raise upper arm outward away from torso until parallel to floor, keeping forearm relaxed in downward "scarecrow" position
Rep motion	4. rotate forearm 180 degrees upwards, keeping upper arm in place, until forearm points towards ceiling 5. exhale and press dumbbell by extending at elbow, straightening arm overhead 6. pause for 1 second and squeeze muscles 7. inhale and reverse steps back to scarecrow start position 8. complete reps stated in worksheet
Swap	9. rest dumbbell on lap and swap hands 10. complete reps for other arm
End	11. place dumbbell on lap for next exercise or replace on rack

Tips

✓ remember to keep your upper arm parallel to the floor
✓ avoid swinging
✓ practice the motion first, then add the weight

Modifications

• if you are struggling to control the weight, try using a lighter 1

Start / End

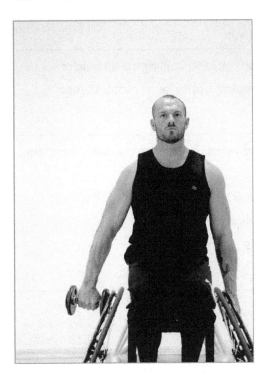

Position 1

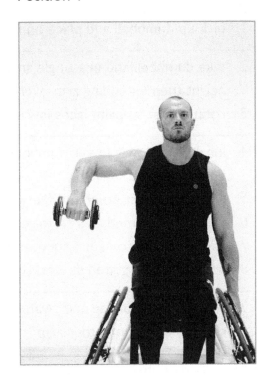

Position 2

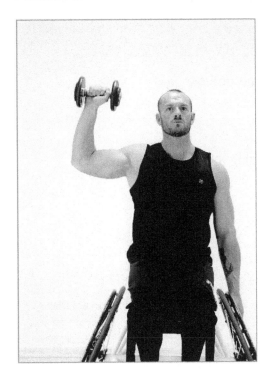

Position 3

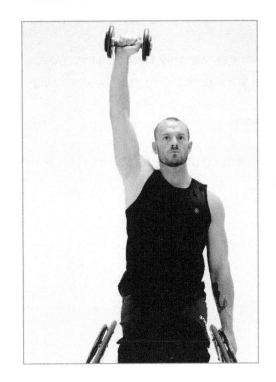

SINGLE-ARM DUMBBELL EXTENSION

Setup	1. pick up dumbbell and place on lap
Start	2. take dumbbell and in a single smooth movement, raising to shoulder height then extending arm overhead keeping upper arm close to ear 3. rotate wrist so palm faces inwards
Rep motion	4. inhale and slowly lower dumbbell behind head, bending at elbow, keeping upper arm still 5. pause at lowest point and feel stretch in triceps 6. exhale and extend arm to raise dumbbell above head 7. pause for 1 second and squeeze muscles 8. complete reps stated in worksheet
Swap	9. rest dumbbell on lap and swap hands 10. complete reps for other arm
End	11. place dumbbell on lap for next exercise or replace on rack

Tips

  ✓ remember it's only the forearm moves
  ✓ keep your upper arm still, next to your head at all times

Modifications

  • if you are struggling to control the weight, try using a lighter 1

Start / End

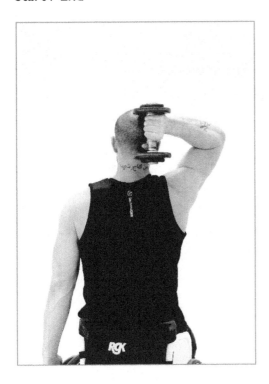

Position 1

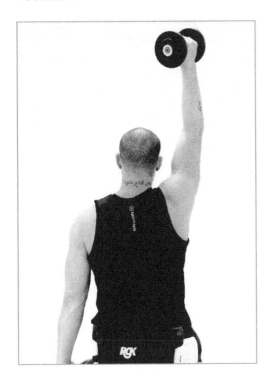

SINGLE-ARM DUMBBELL KICKBACK

Setup	1. pick up dumbbell and place on lap
Start	2. grasp dumbbell in right hand with palms facing torso 3. hold onto an incline bench or chair with left hand for stability 4. keep neutral spine and bend forward at waist until torso almost parallel with floor, keeping head up 5. keep upper arm in and parallel to floor 6. point forearm towards floor so 90-degree angle forms between forearm and upper arm
Rep motion	7. exhale, lift weight and focus on moving forearm until arm is fully extended, keeping upper arm still 8. pause for a second and squeeze muscles 9. inhale and slowly lower dumbbell back down to start position 10. complete reps stated in worksheet
Swap	11. rest dumbbell on lap and swap hands 12. complete reps for other arm
End	13. place dumbbell on lap for next exercise or replace on rack

Start / End

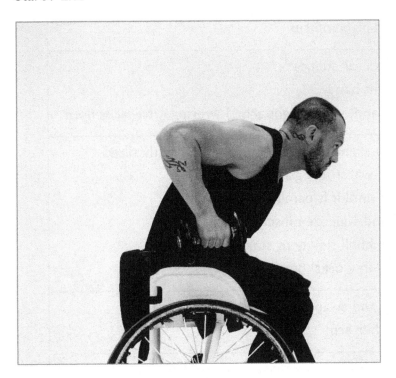

Position 1

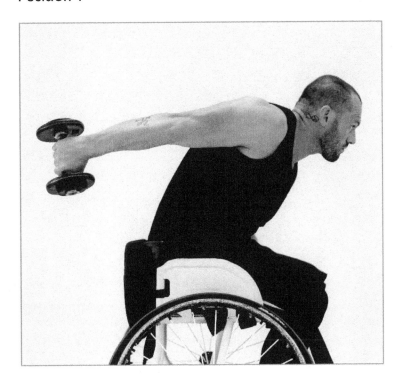

SINGLE-ARM DUMBBELL LAT RAISE

Setup	1. pick up dumbbell and place on lap
Start	2. put left hand on wheel for support
	3. grasp dumbbell in right hand
	4. keep a neutral spine and extend right arm, lowering it towards floor
Rep motion	5. raise dumbbell with a slight bend on elbow, hand slightly tilted forward as if pouring water in a glass
	6. exhale and raise arm until it is parallel to floor
	7. pause for a second and squeeze muscles
	8. inhale and lower dumbbell slowly to start position
	9. complete reps stated in worksheet
Swap	10. rest dumbbell on lap and swap hands
	11. complete reps for other arm
End	12. place dumbbell on lap for next exercise or replace on rack

Tips

✓ remember to avoid swinging

Start / End

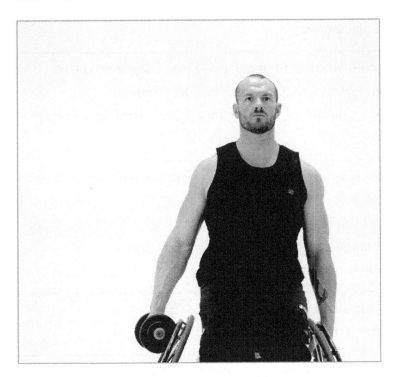

Position 1

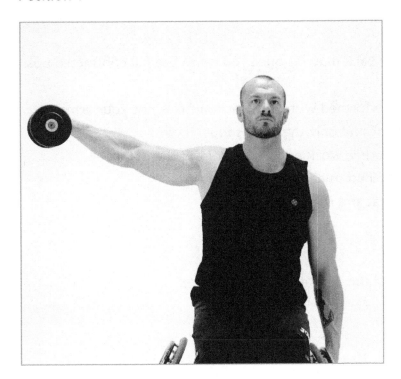

SINGLE-ARM DUMBBELL ROW

Setup	1. pick up dumbbell and place on lap
Start	2. bend torso forward from waist until upper body is 45 degrees to floor, placing left hand on end of incline bench or chair for support 3. use right hand to pick up dumbbell, keeping lower back straight and palm facing torso
Rep motion	4. exhale and pull dumbbell straight up to side of chest, keeping upper arm close to side and torso still 5. pause for a second and squeeze muscles 6. inhale and lower resistance straight down to start position 7. complete reps stated in worksheet
Swap	8. rest dumbbell on lap and swap hands 9. complete reps for other arm
End	10. place dumbbell on lap for next exercise or replace on rack

Tips

- ✓ concentrate on squeezing the back muscles once you reach the full contracted position
- ✓ make sure that the force is performed with your back muscles not your arms
- ✓ upper torso should remain still and only the arms should move
- ✓ your forearms should do no other work except for holding the dumbbell
- ✓ do not try to pull the dumbbell up using the forearms
- ✓ pinch shoulder blades back first and then pull

Modifications

- if you are struggling to control the weight, try using a lighter 1

Start / End

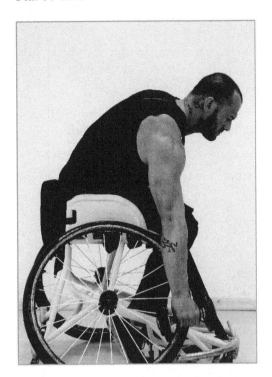

Position 1

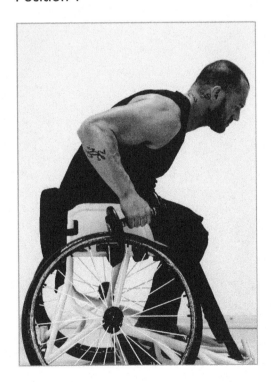

SINGLE-ARM FARMER'S PUSH

Setup	1. pick up dumbbell and place on lap
Start	2. keep back straight and head up 3. grasp dumbbell with left hand and towards floor
Rep motion	4. keep breathing as you do short quick pushes wheel with right hand, moving forwards in a straight line 5. move for a given distance, as fast as possible 6. complete distance stated in worksheet
Swap	7. rest dumbbell on lap and swap hands 8. complete reps for other arm
End	9. place dumbbell on lap for next exercise or replace on rack

Tips

✓ remember to brace to core / trunk whilst doing this

Start

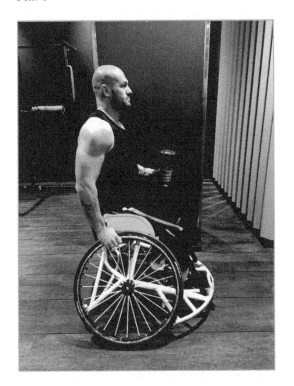

Position 1

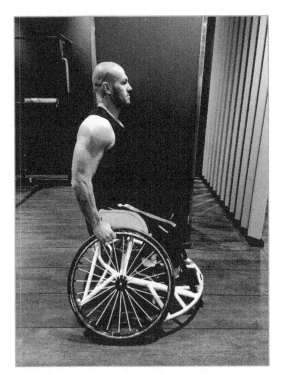

Position 2

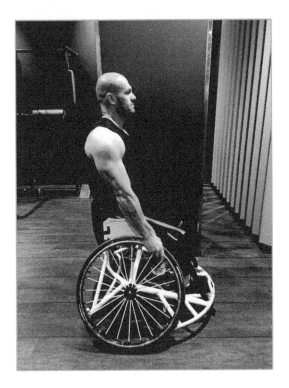

SINGLE-ARM HAMMER CURL

Setup	1. pick up dumbbell and place on lap
Start	2. hold dumbbell in right hand at arm's length, keeping elbows in and palms facing inwards
Rep motion	3. exhale and curl dumbbell upwards, keeping upper arm still and palm facing towards body 4. continue movement until bicep is fully contracted and dumbbell is at shoulder level 5. pause for 1 second and squeeze biceps 6. inhale and slowly lower dumbbell to start position 7. complete reps stated in worksheet
Swap	8. rest dumbbell on lap and swap hands 9. complete reps for other arm
End	10. place dumbbell on lap for next exercise or replace on rack

Tips

✓ remember to only move your forearm

Modifications

• if you are struggling to control the weight, try using a lighter 1

Start / End

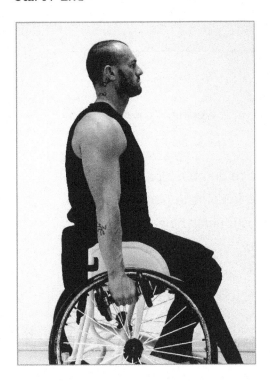

Position 1

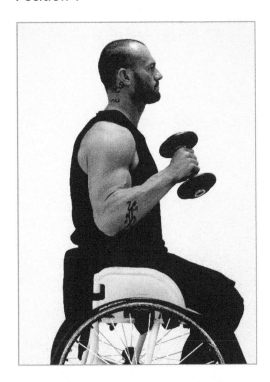

SINGLE-ARM ROTATING CURL

Setup	1. pick up dumbbell and place on lap
Start	2. put left hand on wheel for support 3. grasp dumbbell in right hand 4. keep a neutral spine and extend right arm, lowering it towards floor 5. rotate palm so it faces inwards
Rep motion	6. exhale and curl weight, twisting wrist once dumbbell passes thigh so palm faces forward at end of movement, keeping upper arm still 7. continue movement until dumbbell is at shoulder height 8. pause for 1 second and squeeze muscles 9. inhale and lower dumbbell slowly to start position, rotating wrist so it ends facing inwards 10. complete reps stated in worksheet
Swap	11. rest dumbbell on lap and swap hands 12. complete reps for other arm
End	13. place dumbbell on lap for next exercise or replace on rack

Start / End

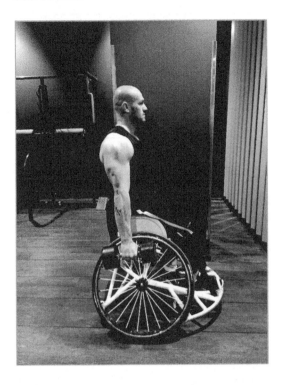

Position 1

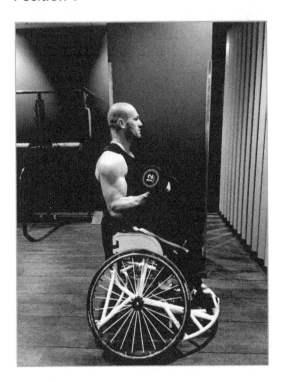

SINGLE-ARM SHOULDER PRESS

Setup	1. pick up dumbbell and place on lap
	2. use left hand to hold onto chair for stability
Start	3. grasp dumbbell with right hand and raise to shoulder height
	4. rotate wrist so palm faces forwards
Rep motion	5. exhale and push dumbbell up until arm is fully extended
	6. pause for a second and squeeze muscles
	7. inhale and lower dumbbell back to start position
	8. complete reps stated in worksheet
Swap	9. rest dumbbell on lap and swap hands
	10. complete reps for other arm
End	11. place dumbbell on lap for next exercise or replace on rack

Tips

✓ remember to avoid locking your elbow joint fully

Start / End

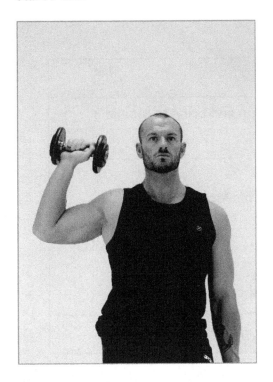

Position 1

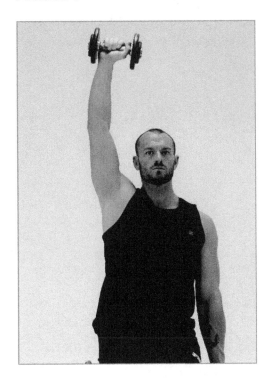

PLATES

CROSSING PLATE PUNCHES

Setup	1. pick up plate and place on lap
Start	2. grasp plate and "3 and 9 o'clock" position and bring to shoulder height
Rep motion	3. keep a neutral spine 4. exhale and explosively fully extended arms forwards 5. return right hand to shoulder 6. maintaining control, switch arm positions as quickly and explosively as possible 7. complete time duration stated in worksheet
End	8. place plate on lap for next exercise or replace on rack

Modifications

Here is slight variation on the plate punch. Instead of moving in and out, add a direction

1. left
2. right
3. up and diagonally to left
4. up and diagonally to right
5. up overhead

This is 1 rep. Repeat for set amount of reps or time.

Start / End

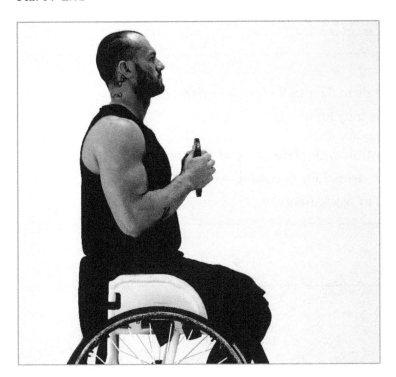

Position 1

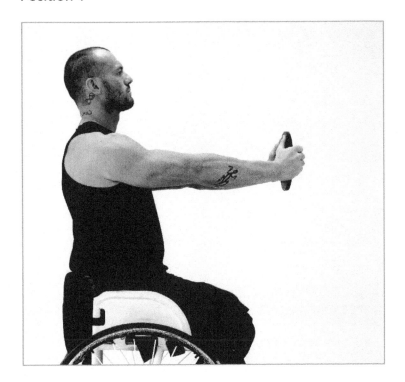

PLATE FIGURE 8S

Setup	1. pick up plate and place on lap
Start	2. keep a neutral spine 3. hold plate in both hands in "3 and 9 o'clock" position 4. raise and extend arms fully forwards
Rep motion	5. make a figure of 8 motion with plate going as high and wide as possible, keeping your arms fully extended whole time 6. complete reps stated in worksheet
End	7. rest plate on lap 8. replace plate

Tips

✓ 1 figure of 8 is a single rep
✓ use a light weight to start with as you don't have a supporting arm with this exercise

Start / End

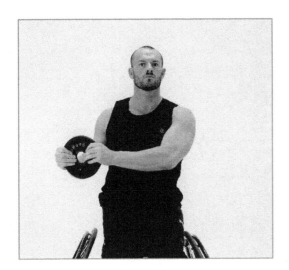

Position 1

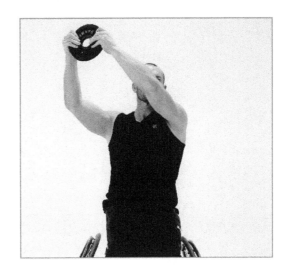

Position 2

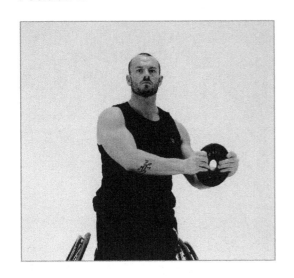

Position 3

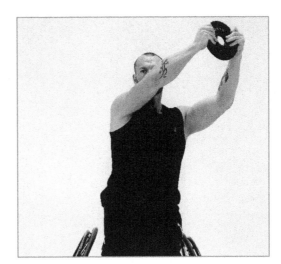

REST AND RECOVERY

When people think about sports performance, be it on the football field, basketball court or in the gym, they tend to think of 2 determining factors after natural ability. These are training and nutrition, usually in that order of importance. Although these 2 things are immensely important, what often gets overlooked is getting adequate rest.

Let's look at what will dramatically improve, not only your performance but your general wellbeing too.

SLEEP

Number 1 on my list is making sure that you get sufficient "quality" sleep each and every night. You must give your central nervous system time to fully recover from the stress that is put upon it daily. Here are some examples of things that cause stress

- training hard
- reduced calories for those that are dieting
- a bad night's sleep the previous night
- a bad day at work
- relationship problems

All of these things are going to affect how you feel physically and mentally. If you're not sleeping well on top of this, it's only a matter of time before you will suffer *overtraining* (also known as burnout.)

HOW TO BOOST SLEEP QUALITY

Here are some easy changes you can make to boost your sleep

- make your bedroom as dark as possible eliminating all light using things like black-out blinds / curtains and eye masks
- no phones or computers at least 1 hour before bed as the blue light emitted by these deivces stops the secretion of melatonin, your sleep hormone, making it harder for you to get off to sleep
- no caffeine after 16.00 – the half-life of caffeine is around 5 hours meaning if you have 200mg of caffeine at 16:00 then at 21:00 you will still have 100mg in your system,

then at 02:00 you will have 50mg and so on (as you know caffeine is a stimulant, making you less tired and more alert)

- magnesium supplements either in pill or topical spray form
- lavender oil can be put onto your pillow or you can get it as a herbal supplement
- melatonin supplements – note this is not permitted in some countries so double check

Bottom line, aim for 7 to 8 hours per night and try and get to bed between 22:00 and 23:00pm... You will know once you start to get quality sleep as you will not need your alarm to wake you in the mornings. Twenty minute power naps during the day, if your schedule allows, are also beneficial.

PRE- AND POST-WORKOUT NUTRITION

There is so much information being thrown about at the moment regarding pre- and post-workout nutrition it can be a little daunting choosing what to do. What is often the most optimal way of doing things can be a chore for the everyday person. A pro-athlete implements the most optimal way of doing things because that is their job. They will probably have more time to think about and do what needs to be done. Having said that, getting a basic pre- and post-workout protocol is pretty easy.

Pre-workout, you want to make sure you have a sufficient amount of protein with either fats, carbohydrates or both. This minimises *muscle catabolism* whilst training which is when your muscles break down. At the very least, if eating is not an option, get some *branch chained amino acids* (BCAAs) protein. In a nutshell, this supplement will stop muscle catabolism. It is available either in drink or tablet form.

> **TIP:** I personally prefer (pre-gym) to have liquid nutrition. This is easier on the digestive system and doesn't make me feel bloated. This could be a shake comprised of oats, whey protein and peanut butter (See my "go to" drink below – it's one of my favourites.)

A go to drink is

- 100g gluten-free oats
- 40g whey protein
- 20g peanut or almond butter

Pre-sports sessions (any performance-based game or event) I prefer a carbohydrate-rich meal around 2 to 3 hours before I play.

Post workout, in all honesty, this totally depends on what type of training you do. For ZART, you should aim for 30 to 40g of protein post workout either in shake form or whole food, whichever you prefer. Whey protein will be absorbed by the body quicker so I would side with that.

Afterwards, eat a protein-rich meal (30 to 40g again) around an hour later. Include a good source of carbs (sweet potatoes, for example) which will ensure you're replenishing glycogen levels. Eating this way means you will be good to go when it's time for the next workout.

MOBILITY AND STRETCHING

The main reason for performing the mobility exercises are to open up your joints, allowing them to move more freely. Key areas to focus on are the

- thoracic (upper) spine
- shoulders (scapulas)
- hips

So many people suffer with lower back pain. If you perform mobility work on a regular basis then you should start to see improvements in this area very quickly.

Mobility exercises should be performed as a warm-up to your workouts and not static stretching. Static stretching pre-training is counter-productive and actually weakens the muscles, making them less powerful and explosive. It also makes them more prone to injury as it weakens them slightly.

Stretching should be performed after training. Regular stretching will increase the range of movement in the muscles you stretch, thus resulting in better performance and reducing your chance of injury. I like to perform a full-body stretching program post-workout but if you have time constraints, focus on the body parts you've just worked.

Mobility work can also be performed as solo sessions, or when you are on your rest days.

FOAM ROLLING AND SELF TRIGGER POINT RELEASE

Foam rolling is self-myofascial release... It's similar to getting a soft-tissue massage from a massage therapist. For example, if you have just trained your chest in the gym, post workout, if you foam roll your chest then you are helping get rid of all the built up lactic acid that's in there. It gets the blood flowing properly. That blood is transporting all the vital nutrients that the muscle will need to repair itself and adapt from the training session you've just had.

> **TIP:** I like to quickly foam roll the working muscle pre-workout. This helps get some blood flowing and open me up a little... rolling should be incorporated into your mobility work too.

EXTRA THINGS THAT CAN REALLY HELP

There are a couple of things to consider to boost your recovery rate

- 5g of creatine as a supplement post workout
- daily high-quality omega 3 supplements will help reduce inflammation and speed up your recovery rate

During periods of high-intensity or high-volume training, taking adaptogenic (physiologically stress-reducing) herbs like

- ashwagandha
- holy basil
- liquorice

help lower cortisol levels, again, allowing for a speedier recovery.

> **TIP:** A great supplement I use for this is CNS Recover from Genetic Supplements.

For boosting sleep quality try

- drinking tulsi tea before bed
- taking Epsom salt baths 1 to 2 times per week

If you can start to implement some of these strategies then you will be on your way to recovering much quicker from the training that you do.

GLOSSARY

Adaptation

This is the process where the body adapts to the training stimulus that you put it under and therefore improves in some way, shape or form.

Adrenal fatigue

The adrenal glands function below the necessary level. Most commonly associated with intense or prolonged stress. Sufferers have fatigue that is not relieved by sleep. People may look and act relatively normal with adrenal fatigue and may not have any obvious signs of physical illness, yet live with a general sense of unwellness.

Avascular necrosis

The death of bone tissue due to a lack of blood supply. It can lead to tiny breaks in the bone and the bone's eventual collapse. The blood flow to a section of bone can be interrupted if the bone is fractured or the joint becomes dislocated.

Branch chained amino acids

Essential amino acids, specifically valine, leucine and isoleucine. They are essential, meaning we must get them in our diet because our bodies can't produce them, only absorb them.

Concentric

The positive or lifting part of the rep, i.e. the lifting of the dumbbell in a bicep curl.

Cortisol

A hormone produced from cholesterol in the 2 adrenal glands lying just above each kidney. It is normally released in response to events and circumstances such as waking up in the morning, exercising, and acute stress.

Creatine monohydrate

A popular supplement used by people looking to build lean muscle mass, maximize performance and increase strength.

Eccentric

The negative or lowering part of the rep, i.e. the lowering of the dumbbell in a bicep curl.

Empty calories

Unlike nutrient-dense foods, which are foods that provide more nutrients than calories, empty-calorie foods contain more calories than nutrients.

Hydrogenated vegetable oil (including trans fats)

Oils (such as vegetable, olive, sunflower) are liquids at room temperature. In the food industry, hydrogen is added to oils (in a process called hydrogenation) to make them more solid, or "spreadable" and also prolong shelf life. The problem with partially hydrogenated oils is that they contain *trans fats*, which raise LDL ("bad") cholesterol, lower HDL ("good") cholesterol and has other harmful effects.

Hypertrophy

The growth and increase of the size of muscle cells. The most common type of muscular hypertrophy occurs because of physical exercise such as weight lifting. The term is often associated with weight training. As you continue to exercise, there is a complex interaction of nervous system responses. This results in an increase in protein synthesis over months and the muscle cells begin to grow larger and stronger.

Lactose intolerant

Adults and children unable to digest lactose are called lactose intolerant. Lactose is a sugar found in milk and to a lesser extent dairy products, causing side effects.

Loading phase

Taking in higher amounts of creatine to saturate or load the muscle with creatine.

Muscle catabolism

Catabolism is the set of metabolic pathways that breaks down molecules into smaller units and reused in the body, in this case muscle tissue.

Overtraining (also known as burnout)

A state that you can get into from too much training, causing enormous stress on the central nervous system without adequate rest and recovery. Symptoms include fatigue, poor exercise performance, frequent upper-respiratory tract infections, altered mood, general malaise, weight loss, muscle stiffness and soreness, and loss of interest in high-level training. (Trust me, you don't ever want to get this, although it is a hard state to get into.)

Periodised

This is when we change the workout protocol on a monthly basis, with a different focus to keep you progressing forwards.

Plateauing

This is when your progress stalls and stagnates. This is why variety is so important. It keeps your body guessing to stop your progress from slowing.

Protein shakes

Protein shakes are drinks made by mixing protein powder with water, although other ingredients are often added as well. They can be a convenient, cost-effective addition to the diet, especially when access to quality high-protein foods is limited.

Superset

A superset is performed when 2 exercises are performed in a row without stopping.

RESOURCES

The downloads are on my ZART website, http://www.zar-training.com. I've included:

- 2 calorie intake needs calculators (1 for gaining muscle and 1 for losing fat)
- meal planner
- shopping list
- training planner workout log
- training methods sheet

KEEP IN TOUCH

I hope you have enjoyed learning about the ZART program with me. I wish you every success. Do share your fitness stories. I'd love to hear from you.

Email them to me at

- dan@zar-training.com

I'd also like to invite you to join my dedicated ZART Facebook group. You're also welcome to join "Feel, Look & Perform Amazing" where I share hints and tips with all my clients.

- https://www.facebook.com/groups/zeroassistance/
- https://www.facebook.com/groups/DanHighcock/

WANT TO ME TO TRAIN YOU

I mentioned that I also love to work with people online so if you're looking for more advice, accountability and support, let me know.

ONE-TO-ONE ZART TRAINING

I also offer a premium personalised 12-week program for chair users who want individual attention as they follow the workouts. Send me an email and let me know you're interested.

To your success,

Dan

Made in United States
Orlando, FL
04 October 2022

23007431R00089